DIFFERENTIAL DIAGNOSIS
IN PATHOLOGY:

GYNECOLOGIC AND OBSTETRICAL DISORDERS

DIFFERENTIAL DIAGNOSIS IN PATHOLOGY

Series Editor: JONATHAN I. EPSTEIN, M.D.

Urologic Disorders
Jonathan I. Epstein, M.D.

Liver Disorders
Swan N. Thung, M.D.
Michael A. Gerber, M.D.

Bone and Joint Disorders
Edward F. McCarthy, M.D.

Breast Disorders
Ayten Someren, M.D.
C. Whitaker Sewell, M.D.

Pulmonary Disorders
Anthony A. Gal, M.D.
Michael N. Koss, M.D.

Vulvar, Vaginal, and Cervical Disorders
W. Dwayne Lawrence, M.D.
Fadi W. Abdul-Karim, M.D.

DIFFERENTIAL DIAGNOSIS IN PATHOLOGY:
GYNECOLOGIC AND OBSTETRICAL DISORDERS

VOLUME I

W. DWAYNE LAWRENCE, M.D.

Chief of Pathology, Hutzel Hospital-Detroit Medical Center
Professor and Director of Anatomic Pathology
Wayne State University School of Medicine
Detroit, Michigan

FADI W. ABDUL-KARIM, M.D.

Director of Anatomic Pathology
Associate Professor of Pathology
Institute of Pathology
Case Western Reserve University School of Medicine
Cleveland, Ohio

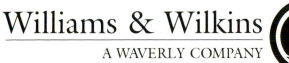

Williams & Wilkins
A WAVERLY COMPANY

SANS TACHE

BALTIMORE • PHILADELPHIA • LONDON • PARIS • BANGKOK
BUENOS AIRES • HONG KONG • MUNICH • SYDNEY • TOKYO • WROCLAW

Editor: Charles W. Mitchell
Marketing Manager: Lorraine A. Smith
Production Coordinator: Dana M. Soares-Jackson
Typesetter: Peirce Graphic Services, Inc.
Printer: Quebecor Printing Book Group

351 West Camden Street
Baltimore, Maryland 21201-2436 USA

Rose Tree Corporate Center
1400 North Providence Road
Building II, Suite 5025
Media, Pennsylvania 19063-2043 USA

Accurate indications, adverse reactions and dosage schedules for drugs are provided in this book, but it is possible that they may change. The reader is urged to review the package information data of the manufacturers of the medications mentioned.

Printed in the United States of America

Library of Congress Cataloging in Publication Data

Lawrence, W. Dwayne.
   Differential diagnosis in pathology : gynecologic and obstetrical disorders / W. Dwayne Lawrence,
     Fadi W. Abdul-Karim. — 1st ed.
     p.   cm. — (Differential diagnosis in pathology.)
   Includes bibliographical references and index.
   ISBN 0-683-30339-2
   1. Gynecologic pathology.   2. Diagnosis, Differential.   I. Abdul-Karim, Fadi.   II. Title.   III. Series.
     [DNLM: 1. Genital Diseases, Female—pathology.   2. Diagnosis, Differential.   WP 141 L424d
     1998]
   RG77.L38   1998
   618.1'07—dc21
   DNLM/DLC
   for Library of Congress   97-50435
                                                                                                        CIP

First Edition,

The publishers have made every effort to trace the copyright holders for borrowed material. If they have inadvertently overlooked any, they will be pleased to make the necessary arrangements at the first opportunity.

To purchase additional copies of this book, call our customer service department at **(800) 638-0672** or fax orders to **(800) 447-8438**. For other book services, including chapter reprints and large quantity sales, ask for the Special Sales department.

Canadian customers should call **(800) 665-1148,** or fax **(800) 665-0103.** For all other calls originating outside of the United States, please call **(410) 528-4223** or fax us at **(410) 528-8550.**

Visit Williams & Wilkins on the Internet: **http://www.wwilkins.com** or contact our customer service department at **custserv@wwilkins.com.** Williams & Wilkins customer service representatives are available from 8:30 am to 6:00 pm, EST, Monday through Friday, for telephone access.

98 99 00
1 2 3 4 5 6 7 8 9 10

PREFACE

The books comprising the **Differential Diagnoses in Surgical Pathology** series follow a uniform format that is somewhat different from the standard textbooks in surgical pathology, in that two or more specific differential diagnoses in a particular organ system are discussed and illustrated together. To preserve economy of space, the explanations for the figures are incorporated within the text. The book is largely morphologically-oriented, therefore, a great majority of the figures are black and white photomicrographs of standard H&E sections accompanied by some pertinent gross photographs. The bibliography, as in the previous volumes of this series, has been restricted to a relatively few important references within which the reader can find more in-depth discussion as well as a more extensive bibliography for further study.

This particular volume deals with Gynecologic Disorders of the Lower Female Genital Tract, including the vulva, vagina, and cervix. It is certainly not intended to supplant the more detailed and comprehensive textbooks of gynecologic pathology that are currently available, but rather to provide an ancillary tool to aid further in the differential diagnosis of confusing gynecologic disorders. An attempt has been made to confine the chapters largely to lesions which the surgical pathologist might encounter in daily practice; however, more unusual lower female genital tract entities have been included when the possibility of their confusion with other diagnostic entities, either benign or malignant, has important clinical consequences to the patient.

It is our wish that this book will prove helpful to pathologists-in-training, practicing surgical pathologists, and clinicians having a special interest in gynecologic pathology, with the ultimate goal of insuring that patients receive, foremost, a correct diagnosis and, consequently, proper treatment.

W. Dwayne Lawrence, M.D.
Detroit, Michigan
Fadi W. Abdul-Karim, M.D.
Cleveland, Ohio

DEDICATION

Charles S. Lawrence
William Abdul-Karim

ACKNOWLEDGMENTS

We are grateful to our pathology colleagues, fellows, and residents in our respective departments for contributing on a daily basis to the stimulating and collegial environment that has enabled our continued professional growth. We acknowledge our appreciation to the following pathologists who have provided us with examples of some of the illustrated entities herein: Drs. Robert E. Scully, Lyn M. Duncan, and Judith A. Ferry at the Massachusetts General Hospital and Harvard Medical School, Dr. George Murphy at Thomas Jefferson University Hospital, Dr. Phyllis C. Huettner at Washington University Medical Center, and Drs. Raymond Redline, Joseph E. Willis, and Caroline Steinetz at the Institute of Pathology, Case Western Reserve University School of Medicine. We are also grateful to Ms. Christine MacKay, Ms. Amber Baumgardner, and Ms. Doris Willis for their assistance in preparing the manuscript.

CONTENTS

SECTION 1: VULVAR DISORDERS

SECTION 2: VAGINAL DISORDERS

SECTION 3: CERVICAL DISORDERS

Section 1   VULVAR DISORDERS

1. Non-neoplastic Epithelial Disorders: Lichen Sclerosus vs. Lichen Simplex Chronicus vs. Squamous Cell Hyperplasia

CLINICAL

The International Society of Gynecological Pathologists (ISGP), the International Society of Vulvar Disease (ISSVD), and the World Health Organization (WHO) have approved the following classification of non-neoplastic epithelial disorders (NNEDs; formerly "vulvar dystrophies") : i) Lichen sclerosus (LS) ii) Squamous cell hyperplasia (SCH), not otherwise specified (NOS), and iii) other dermatoses, of which lichen simplex chronicus (LSC) is probably the most common. LS represents 30–40% of all NNEDs and manifests somewhat more distinctive clinical and pathologic features than either LSC or SCH. LS usually affects the vulva and perineum of perimenopausal and postmenopausal women, and the most commonly encountered sites include the labia minora, the labia majora, the clitoris, the perineum, and the posterior fourchette in descending order of frequency. Lesions are pruritic, multifocal, and often symmetrical. LS patients have a higher incidence of autoimmune-related diseases than the general population, and some cases may be familial.

LSC is also common (representing 20–30% of NNEDs) and many workers have included it under the rubric of SCH; however, the clinicopathologic features of LSC are sufficiently distinctive to regard it as a separate dermatosis. Therefore, vulvar SCH NOS ("hyperplastic dystrophy") in its typical form is infrequently encountered. About two-thirds of women with LSC and SCH are premenopausal, although both may afflict postmenopausal women. Favored sites include the labia majora and mons, the outer labia minora, the clitoral hood and the interlabial sulci. LSC and SCH are generally considered to represent a nonspecific response to chronic irritation and many cases of vulvar SCH AND LSC, but particularly the latter, likely represent the lesion previously designated as "neurodermatitis".

LS, LSC and SCH may affect separate or contiguous areas on the same vulva; alternatively, the changes of SCH may be superimposed on LS ("mixed dystrophies"), such combinations representing about 15% of NNEDs. However, when combined NNEDs occur, the ISGP, the ISSVD, and the WHO recommend reporting each as a separate diagnosis.

GROSS

Early lesions of LS are characterized by multiple, pale pink to white papules that coalesce to form well-delineated, roughened white plaques. Melanin incontinence into the dermis may less commonly impart a brown discoloration to some lesions. In advanced LS, the vulvar skin and mucosa are thin and atrophic, appearing dry and exhibiting a parchment-like or "cigarette paper" effect. Because of atrophy and the frequently associated pruritus with consequent rubbing and scratching, telangiectasias and ecchymoses are often present. There is progressive resorption of the labia, particularly the labia minora. The latter may become agglutinated and, along with the clitoris, disappear completely. Vulvar tissues undergo extensive contracture, and in far advanced cases severe stenosis of the introitus occurs.

LSC is often associated with lichenification, a thickening of the skin with prominence and accentuation of skin markings, secondary to itching and rubbing. A white component is often present.

Early lesions of SCH may also begin as discrete pink to red or white plaques that may or may not be multiple. SCH lesions are infrequently symmetrical and resorption and dissolution of the labia are rarely present. The gross appearance of both LSC and SCH is usually dependent on the degree of upper epidermal or mucosal keratinization; the greater the latter, the white the lesion. Lichenification is a regularly encountered feature of both. Excoriations may occur.

Anogenital mixed NNEDs exhibit either classic findings of each on separate or contiguous areas, or of one superimposed on the other; the latter is most commonly represented by SCH or LSC superimposed on LS. A prominent white surface change associated with vulvar atrophy and contracture points toward a mixed NNED.

HISTOPATHOLOGY

Early LS is characterized by a squamous epithelium of normal or mildly hyperplastic thickness; however, the dermal changes, which are pathognomonic of LS, are already apparent. The dermis is edematous and exhibits the superficial band of hyalinized abnormal collagen, which is the hallmark of LS (Fig. 1.1). Superficial vessels of the papillary dermis are telangiectatic (Fig. 1.2). Progressive lesions of LS show increasing degrees of squamous epithelial atrophy with blunting, flattening, and loss of rete pegs (Fig. 1.3). Sweat glands and pilosebaceous units gradually disappear. Although there is progressive thinning of the squamous epithelium (Fig. 1.4), hyperkeratosis or parakeratosis may be prominent, probably depending on the amount of associated rubbing and scratching. Intraepithelial melanin pigment in the form of melanocytes and keratinocytes containing melanosomes markedly decreases, contributing, along with the hyperkeratosis and parakeratosis (Fig. 1.5), to the degree of whiteness of the lesion. However, there may be considerable melanin incontinence into the dermis. In some cases with either little or no hyperkeratosis, the latter may impart the aforementioned brown pigmentation to LS. There may be focally prominent hydropic and vacuolar degenerative changes at the epithelial-dermal junction (Fig. 1.6). These may result in subepidermal bullae and consequent epidermal denudation.

The dermis in advanced LS shows a progressive diminution in cellularity in the characteristic hyalinized band-like zone, along with obliteration of the previously ectatic vascular lumens in the papillary dermis. The subepithelial bullae may separate from the dermis, and the subsequent picture may raise the question of bullous skin disease. Special stains usually will show elastic fibers to be markedly decreased in numbers in LS (Fig. 1.7). A chronic inflammatory infiltrate, predominantly lymphocytic, is often found subjacent to the band-like hyalinized zone (Fig. 1.8).

Compared to LS, the histopathologic findings in LSC and SCH are somewhat less specific. The squamous epithelium in LSC shows prominent psoriasiform epidermal hyperplasia with acanthosis (Fig. 1.9), hypergranulosis, compact orthokeratosis, and focal parakeratosis. Rete ridges are of unequal width and breadth (Fig. 1.10). The latter may be irregularly thickened and widened, elongated, and sometimes confluent, and are often either pointed or club-shaped (Fig. 1.10). There is relatively regular and orderly maturation with reactive appearing but uniform nuclei. The thickened papillary dermis in LSC shows laminated, coarse bundles of collagen ("vertical streaking of collagen" or "lamellar fibrosis") (Fig. 1.11) and blood vessels, both oriented parallel to the rete. The papillary dermis contains an often prominent superficial chronic inflammatory (usually lymphohistiocytic) infiltrate accompanied by melanophages. SCH

exhibits an even more nonspecific squamous hyperplasia, with hyperkeratosis and parakeratosis, and the microscopic features are emphasized in Chapter 2 (Figs. 2.1–2.3). Mitoses are confined to the basal/parabasal layer, and abnormal forms are not evident. The findings within the dermis are relatively nonspecific, and vertical streaking of collagen is less prominent to absent. Chronic inflammation is likewise mild to absent. In mixed NNEDs, the histopathologic findings are represented (1) by the aforementioned classic findings in either geographically separate or contiguous LS and SCH or (2) more characteristic dermal findings of LS accompanied by overlying epithelial changes more indicative of LSC or SCH in those cases in which a single lesion manifests more than one NNED (Fig. 1.12).

PROGNOSIS AND TREATMENT

LS is commonly observed adjacent to vulvar intraepithelial neoplasia (VIN) and squamous cell carcinoma. Although many workers consider pure LS to have a low malignant potential, some investigators have challenged that supposition and the matter is currently considered controversial. However, since many of the NNEDs, VINs, and invasive squamous cancers tend to present as white lesions, rendering a reliable diagnosis on clinical examination alone may be virtually impossible. Therefore, close follow-up with accurate documentation of appearance, and biopsies as indicated, particularly of any lesion that changes over time, are imperative to preclude the rare development of carcinoma. LS is a chronic, recurring disease marked by progressive atrophy of the vulvar and perivulvar tissues and often intense pruritus. The current mainstay of therapy for most patients is topical testosterone or progesterone and antipruritic medication; treatment may be followed by varying degrees of vulvar restitution.

Patients with LSC and SCH should be followed with the same care and clinical attention as LS patients. Treatment of patients with LSC or SCH begins with removal of the source of irritation followed by treatment with topical corticosteroids and antipruritics.

Mixed NNEDs are treated in the same manner as the individual lesions alone; however, some clinicians will treat the SCH initially, followed by treatment of LS after resolution of the former. Since some feel that mixed NNEDs may have a greater propensity to develop VIN and invasive squamous carcinoma than either NNED alone, such patients must be carefully monitored.

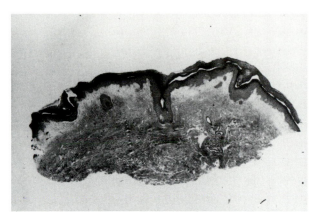

Figure 1.1. Vulvar lichen sclerosus.

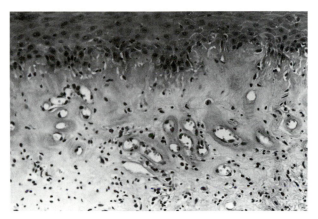

Figure 1.2. Vulvar lichen sclerosus.

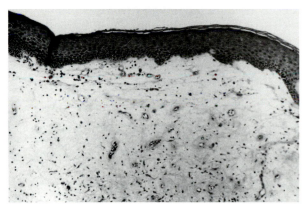

Figure 1.3. Vulvar lichen sclerosus.

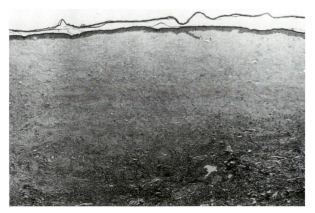

Figure 1.4. Vulvar lichen sclerosus.

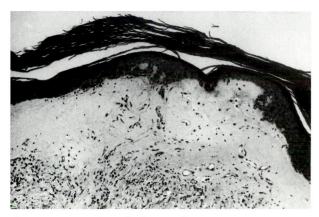

Figure 1.5. Vulvar lichen sclerosus.

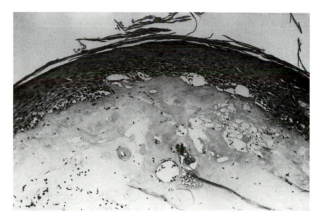

Figure 1.6. Vulvar lichen sclerosus.

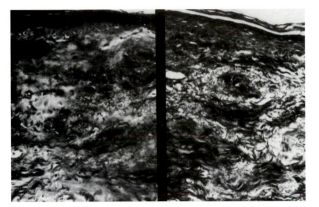

Figure 1.7. Vulvar lichen sclerosus, left; adjacent normal squamous epithelium, right. Elastic stain.

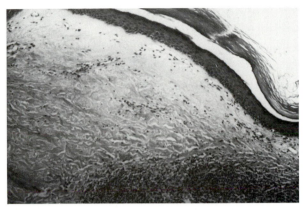

Figure 1.8. Vulvar lichen sclerosus.

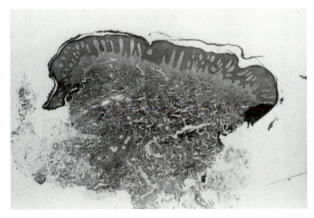

Figure 1.9. Vulvar lichen simplex chronicus.

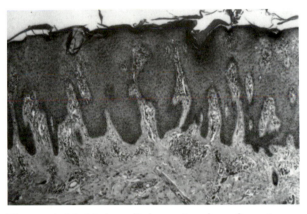

Figure 1.10. Vulvar lichen simplex chronicus.

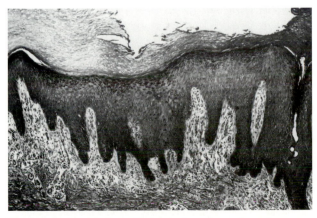

Figure 1.11. Vulvar lichen simplex chronicus.

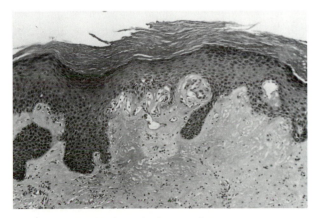

Figure 1.12. Vulvar lichen sclerosus & squamous cell hyperplasia.

2. Non-Neoplastic Epithelial Disorders: Squamous Cell Hyperplasia and Lichen Simplex Chronicus vs. Vulvar Intraepithelial Neoplasia

CLINICAL

The clinical, gross, and treatment and prognostic features of the non-neoplastic epithelial disorders (NNEDs) including lichen simplex chronicus (LSC) and squamous cell hyperplasia (SCH) were discussed in Chapter 1. About 10% of women with either LSC or SCH will have an associated vulvar intraepithelial neoplasia (VIN).

Before 1970, VIN occurred most frequently in women in their fifth and sixth decades; however, currently half of patients are less than 40. Furthermore, half of the latter group have other lower genital tract intraepithelial neoplastic lesions, especially cervical. Younger women tend to have multiple lesions, whereas older patients are more likely to have solitary ones. Although most VIN lesions are asymptomatic, many patients complain of pruritus. The labia minora and perineum seem to be especially susceptible to VIN, and the anal skin and its mucosa are the most frequently involved secondary sites.

GROSS

Like the NNEDs, VIN has a variable gross presentation, at times appearing as discrete or coalescent papules or macules. Seventy per cent of VIN lesions are said to be multifocal, and they typically are raised above the surrounding skin or mucosa, although lower grades of VIN tend to be flatter than higher-grade ones. Approximately half of VINs are white lesions, but the rest may show a red, brown to black, or bluish coloration. About a third of VIN lesions are hyperpigmented; indeed, such represent the second most common cause of vulvar "dark" lesions. Some may be scaly or eczematoid and mimic a dermatosis, whereas others mimic otherwise typical condyloma.

HISTOPATHOLOGY

Although the microscopic features of the NNEDs were discussed in Chapter 1, the illustrations of SCH are emphasized in this chapter. The squamous epithelium of the NNEDs is typified by an acanthotic squamous mucosa, with orderly and progressive maturation as shown by the example of SCH in Figs. 2.1 and 2.2. Mitotic features are seen only in the basal layer. Nuclei are uniform and round to oval with finely dispersed chromatin. Intercellular bridges are distinct (Fig. 2.2). The rete pegs are often club-shaped or elongated with widening and confluence (Fig. 2.2). Hyperkeratosis is a common finding, often joined by parakeratosis (Fig. 2.3) and hypergranulosis. Although the dermis often contains a chronic inflammatory infiltrate, the latter may be sparse to absent in SCH (Figs. 2.1 and 2.2). Low grade VIN is characterized by cells showing a greater degree of crowding than either LSC or SCH, especially in the basal and parabasal layers (Fig. 2.4). The squamous cells overlying the latter show somewhat more orderly maturation as they approach the surface, but nucleocytoplasmic ratios are still higher than in reactive squamous intraepithelial atypias. Nuclei show mild to moderate pleomorphism. Coarsely clumped chromatin and mitotic figures are more frequent (Fig. 2.5) and sometimes abnormal, especially in the lower third of the epithelium. Abnormal mitoses are nearly always seen in VIN and are generally more common with increasing degrees of squamous atypicality. Some workers feel that their absence should at least cast doubt on whether the lesion is a true example of VIN.

Like the NNEDs (LSC & SCH) VIN lesions often show a variably prominent white component that is manifested microscopically by correspondingly variable degrees of hyperkeratosis and parakeratosis. Unlike the NNEDs, VIN lesions may extend into the outer portions of the hair follicles. As previously mentioned, low-grade VIN tends to be a flat lesion and often shows true koilocytosis or koilocytotic atypia (Fig. 2.6) as a reflection of its genesis from human papilloma virus. In fact, some workers prefer to restrict the diagnosis of VIN I to such flat lesions (Fig. 2.6), designating the exophytic variant of the same lesion as condyloma acuminatum. The finding of pure VIN I is a relatively uncommon phenomenon and even most VIN II lesions are seen in association with, or adjacent to, VIN III.

PROGNOSIS AND TREATMENT

Only 2–10% of reported cases of VIN III have progressed to invasive cancer and the progression rate of low-grade VIN, and even VIN II is even lower. Historically, those at greatest risk for invasive cancer were postmenopausal and severely immunosuppressed women. However, relatively recent studies have indicated a disturbing increase in the incidence and prevalence of VIN as well as a concomitant propensity for invasion in premenopausal women; such biological changes may reflect the finding of high-risk HPV serotypes in their lesions. Currently, conservative wide local excision of high-grade VIN is still the treatment of choice; others include laser ablation and skinning vulvectomy. Emphasis is placed on early detection and treatment of VIN lesions, given their accessibility and curability.

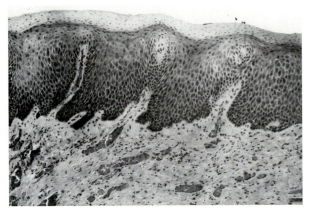

Figure 2.1. Vulvar squamous cell hyperplasia.

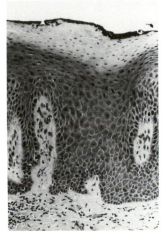

Figure 2.2. Vulvar squamous cell hyperplasia.

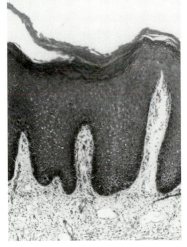

Figure 2.3. Vulvar squamous cell hyperplasia.

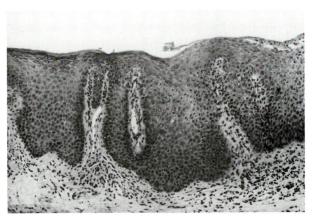

Figure 2.4. Low grade VIN.

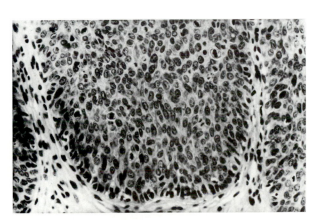

Figure 2.5. Low grade VIN.

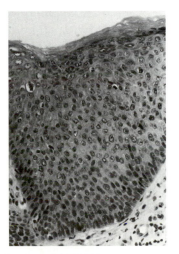

Figure 2.6. Low grade VIN.

3. Reactive and Inflammatory Squamous Mucosal Atypias

vs.

Invasive Squamous Cell Carcinoma

CLINICAL

The reactive and inflammatory squamous mucosal atypias include a widely diverse group of lesions that may be confused with invasive squamous cell carcinoma (SCC). The prototypes that will be discussed in this chapter include lymphogranuloma venereum (LGV), caused by *Chlamydia trachomatis,* and granuloma inguinale (GI), caused by *Calymmatobacterium donovani.* Both are venereally transmitted diseases that are often confused with one another.

Although LGV and GI are relatively unusual, a discussion of their distinction from invasive SCC is warranted, given the serious medical and psychosocial implications of their misdiagnosis.

GROSS

The later stages of LVG and GI are marked by tumor-like masses and distortion of vulvar and perivulvar architecture (Fig. 3.1). Biopsies of such are often are sent with the clinical suspicion of SCC since the latter may present with clinical features similar to those of LGV and GI. Also, so-called postgranulomatous SCCs that rarely arise from longstanding chronic diseases such as LGV and GI are often very large, exophytic tumors.

HISTOPATHOLOGY

Prototypical LGV and GI tend to ulcerate with an adjacent and often marked pseudoepitheliomatous squamous cell hyperplasia (PSCH). Both LGV and GI show relatively nonspecific changes within the ulcer, including a marked chronic inflammatory infiltrate in its base, foci of necrosis sometimes bordered by palisaded epithelioid cells and multinucleated giant cells, dermal fibrosis, lymphangiectasia, and active or healed vasculitis. The causative organisms may be demonstrated in both ulcers by special techniques. The adjacent squamous mucosa of the expanding ulcer may show a markedly atypical PSCH that can be easily mistaken for carcinoma.

The appearance of PSCH present in the ulceronodular and granulomatous lesions of LGV and GI is similar; often elongate, thin, and irregularly shaped rete pegs frequently reach deep into the underlying dermis; however, some pegs may appear bulbous and may mimic either well-dif-

ferentiated ("verrucoid") SCC or verrucous carcinoma (Fig. 3.2). Tangential sections of hyperkeratotic epithelium entrapped in the stroma by the surrounding proliferating squamous epithelium may simulate keratinization within a SCC (Fig. 3.3). Such may also result in irregular islands of quite atypical squamous epithelium that simulate nests of overtly invasive SCC (Fig. 3.4); however, deeper cuts will show that they are connected to the overlying epithelium. Squamous cell nuclei are enlarged, and vesicular and nucleoli may be prominent. Consequently, the distinction from the differentiated type of VIN III (Fig. 3.5) and its corresponding variant of well-differentiated vulvar SCC may be difficult; both in situ and invasive components (Fig. 3.5) are characterized by relatively normal intermediate and superficial layers, sometimes with only mild nuclear atypicality at most, and the basal layers have prominent eosinophilic cytoplasm. Lower-third epithelium nuclei are enlarged and vesicular with dispersed chromatin and prominent nucleoli. Such an architectural and cytologic picture adjacent to an ulcer should make one wary of making the diagnosis of well-differentiated SCC. The presence of so-called stromal changes, manifested by loosening of the connective tissues, edema, and a surrounding chronic inflammatory infiltrate, may also aid in the distinction of SCC from PSCH. Also, the presence of single, invading cells and small nests of tumor can be of some help in identifying carcinoma (Fig. 3.6). Conversely, some SCCs tend to ulcerate, so an ulcerated SCC should not be underdiagnosed. The distinction between PSCH and well-differentiated SCC should be readily evident in most cases, particularly when the lesion is carefully examined microscopically and consideration is given to the surrounding milieu. However, in rare cases their certain distinction is impossible.

PROGNOSIS AND THERAPY

Over time, LGV and GI result in distortion, mutilation, and scarring of the genital skin and mucosa. GI typically remains localized to the presenting area. The late stages of LGV are characterized by rectal and perineal stricture and sometimes draining sinuses. In women, spread of the disease is generally to the deep pelvic and perirectal lymph nodes, the enlargement of which further reinforces the resemblance to cancer. Both LGV and GI respond to appropriate antibiotic therapy.

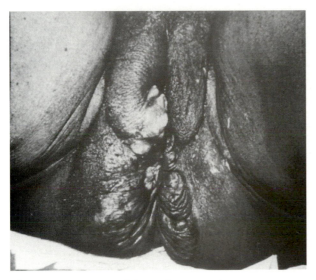

Figure 3.1. Genital lymphogranuloma venereum.

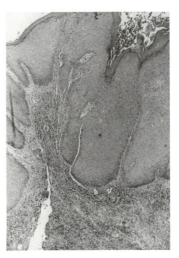

Figure 3.2. Pseudoepitheliomatous hyperplasia-lymphogranuloma venereum.

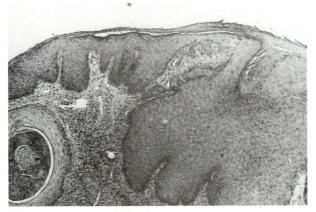

Figure 3.3. Pseudoepitheliomatous hyperplasia-lymphogranuloma venereum.

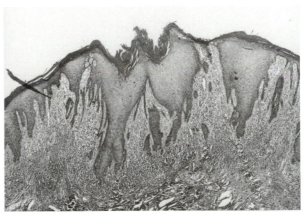

Figure 3.4. Pseudoepitheliomatous hyperplasia-lymphogranuloma venereum.

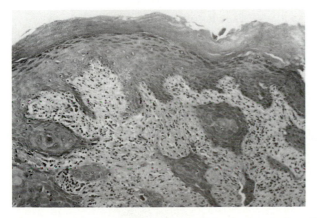

Figure 3.5. Well differentiated superficially invasive squamous cell carcinoma, arising from differentiated VIN III.

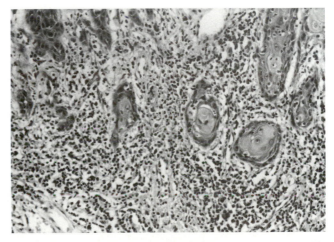

Figure 3.6. Well differentiated superficially invasive squamous cell carcinoma.

4. Granular Cell Tumor

vs.

Invasive Squamous Cell Carcinoma

CLINICAL

Approximately 7% of all granular cell tumors (GCTs) are encountered in the vulvas of young and middle-aged women. Typically slow-growing, they may enlarge rapidly in early pregnancy and cause confusion with squamous cell carcinoma (SCC). Depigmentation and ulceration of overlying skin may also heighten the clinical suspicion for an early SCC.

About 75% of vulvar cancer patients present with a solitary tumor mass, most frequently on the labia majora or minora. Pruritus and ulceration are common. Currently, there is a trend toward a younger age at detection, a concomitant diminution in the size of initially detected SCCs, and an increase in the proportion of early, superficially invasive carcinomas.

GROSS

GCTs are usually relatively small, generally <3 cm in diameter. On cut section, they are discrete but unencapsulated, pale gray to yellow tan, and may be mistaken grossly for a xanthoma.

The gross appearance of SCCs is highly variable, and they may form either an endophytic or exophytic mass; the former may exist either as indurated plaque-like tumors or as excavated lesions with heaped-up, rolled edges. Exophytic tumors may exhibit a fungating, condylomatous, or verrucous appearance or take the form of irregularly nodular excrescences.

HISTOPATHOLOGY

The GCT consists of large, round to polygonal cells with granular, slightly eosinophilic cytoplasm, although the appearance of the latter may be influenced by processing, fixation, and staining. Variably-sized PAS positive-diastase-resistant granules fill the cytoplasm and nuclei are relatively small, uniform, and bland-appearing. Mitotic activity is unusual. GCTs grow as nests, strands, and individual cells at varying depths in the underlying dermis or mucosal stroma. A histopathologic hallmark associated with GCTs is an overlying pseudoepitheliomatous squamous cell hyperplasia (PSCH) (Fig. 4.1) that may mimic well-differentiated SCC. Although PSCH may accompany more than 30 skin diseases, in about two-thirds of GCTs the overlying squamous mucosa shows a downgrowth into the dermis of irregular, elongated, branching rete pegs of variable depth and irregular architecture; because of the latter, sectioning may result in the formation of isolated, irregularly shaped squamous nests and squamous pearls in the dermis or stroma, which raise the question of nests of invasive well-differentiated SCC (Figs. 4.2 and 4.3). However, militating against that diagnosis are the lack of significant nuclear atypicality and sparse mitotic figures. Most PSCH is confined to the papillary dermis, but the biopsy must be sufficiently deep to include the GCT and thus exclude a SCC.

The irregularly infiltrating pattern of a small keratinizing well-differentiated SCC of the vulva is more likely to be confused with the PSCH associated with GCT. In the former, there are abundant eosinophilic cytoplasm, prominent intercellular junctions, frequent pearl formation and infrequent mitotic activity. The invading nests of well-differentiated SCC often, even on low-power examination (Fig. 4.4), show more copious eosinophilic cytoplasm than in the overlying epithelium from which they arise; they may appear to "drop off" the basal aspect of an overlying squamous epithelium that only appears atypical (Fig. 4.4). The irregular shapes of such nests and absence of palisading at their periphery is typical. Intraepithelial squamous pearls may be adjacent to the infiltrating nests in the region of invasion (Fig. 4.5). In contrast to the nuclei seen with the usual PSCH, such nuclei show mild to moderate atypicality. Invasive nests of SCC often exhibit a stromal reaction at their periphery consisting of either loosening or desmoplasia, sometimes accompanied by a variably dense round cell infiltrate (Fig. 4.5). True vascular space invasion is a feature seen in invasive SCC in contrast to such an appearance in the stromal PSCH associated with a granular cell tumor; the latter more likely would be due to a tangentially sectioned squamous nest surrounded by a clear space, representing retraction artifact engendered by tissue processing. However, it should be noted that the degree of PSCH may be so marked that unequivocal distinction from a well-differentiated SCC may be very difficult or impossible in a superficial biopsy (Fig. 4.6: left panel, GCT; right panel, SCC).

PROGNOSIS AND TREATMENT

Virtually all GCTs are benign and do not recur after adequate wide local surgical excision; however, they may infiltrate locally and recur if incompletely removed. Therapy for SCC is different from that of GCT, so misdiagnosis may lead to radical overtreatment. Many institutions individualize treatment for vulvar SCC so that small stage I tumors with superficial invasion are treated less aggressively whereas tumors ≥2 cm in diameter (stage III) receive more radical therapy. Misdiagnosis of PSCH associated with a larger GCT of stage II size could result in serious and disfiguring overtreatment with potentially damaging consequences.

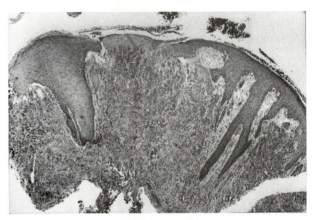

Figure 4.1. Granular cell tumor.

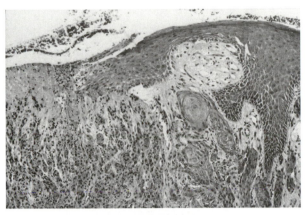

Figure 4.2. Granular cell tumor with ulceration.

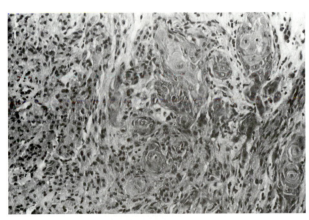

Figure 4.3. Granular cell tumor.

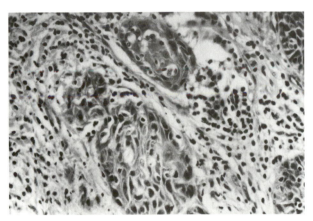

Figure 4.4. Superficially invasive well differentiated squamous cell carcinoma.

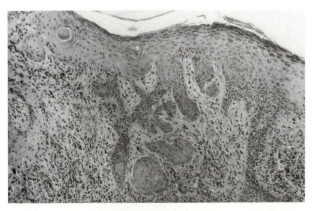

Figure 4.5. Superficially invasive well differentiated squamous cell carcinoma.

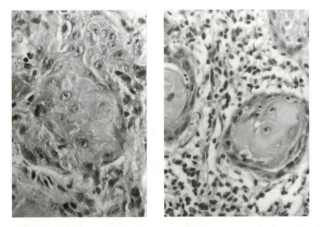

Figure 4.6. Granular cell tumor, left; Well differentiated squamous cell carcinoma, right.

5. Vulvar Intraepithelial Neoplasia vs. "Bowenoid Papulosis" vs. Intraepithelial Squamous Atypia from Podophyllin Effect

CLINICAL

The clinical aspects of vulvar intraepithelial neoplasia (VIN) are covered in Chapter 2.

So-called "bowenoid papulosis" (BP) has generated considerable controversy over the last two decades, and most internationally sanctioned committees on nomenclature no longer recommend its use. Lesions that have been designated as "BP" most often occur in young women between the ages of 20 and 40. About 10% of reported patients have been pregnant. Two-thirds of the lesions of "BP" are multiple and commonly extensive, involving the labia minora and inner labia majora, the introitus, the vagina, the urethra, and even the anal canal. Patients may complain of pruritus.

Podophyllin (POD) is a resinous mixture containing a cytotoxic agent that has a colchicine-like effect on rapidly proliferating tissues. POD most effectively treats the small, newly formed warts of condyloma acuminata, in which regression is most likely to occur. It has little effect on nonvenereally transmitted warts or on older, established flat lesions of condyloma.

The appearance of squamous lesions of the vulva after POD application is well known to mimic the cytologic changes of VIN and confuse their microscopic interpretation. These effects often diminish within 2 weeks after the last application but may persist for up to a month or more.

GROSS

The gross features of VIN are covered in Chapter 2; note that the pigmented high-grade VINs grossly may mimic a variety of other vulvar skin disorders, including not only benign diseases such as nonneoplastic epithelial disorders, condylomata, nevi, hemangiomas, and seborrheic keratoses, but also malignant ones such as melanoma and extramammary Paget's disease.

The lesions clinically diagnosed as "BP" often appear as slightly elevated papules (Fig. 5.1), varying from tan to red-brown or even blue or violet in color, which may become confluent to form small plaques. The usually multiple lesions of "BP" may be confused with other venere-ally transmitted diseases such as condyloma acuminatum and molluscum contagiosum.

Condylomata treated with POD show no distinctive gross features, although the extensive necrosis that may be seen in larger lesions might simulate invasive squamous cancer. However, since smaller condylomata are optimal candidates for POD therapy, it is their microscopic examination that usually engenders the question of VIN.

HISTOPATHOLOGY

Proliferative squamous intraepithelial lesions of the vulvar epidermis or squamous mucosa formerly classified as mild and moderate squamous dysplasia are currently placed into VIN I and VIN II categories, respectively; severe squamous dysplasia and carcinoma in situ combine to form VIN III. VIN lesions exhibit varying degrees of maturational abnormality manifested by both architectural and cytologic atypicality. Cytologic abnormalities include diminution in cytoplasmic volume; nuclear enlargement; increased nucleocytoplasmic ratio, coarsening and clumping of nuclear chromatin, increased mitotic activity with abnormal forms (Figs. 5.2, 5.4), irregularity of the nuclear membrane, and nuclear pleomorphism. "Architectural" abnormalities are manifested primarily by the level of the epithelium replaced by the aforementioned atypical and neoplastic squamous cells; the cells overlying them, however, usually exhibit greater, albeit abnormal, degrees of maturation or differentiation.

VIN I lesions show the foregoing changes primarily in the lower third epithelium (Fig. 5.3), and mitotic figures are confined to the basal and parabasal layers with orderly maturation above them. VIN I lesions are most often flat and exhibit koilocytotic nuclear atypicality (Fig. 5.3). Some workers, therefore, refer to them as flat condylomas of the vulva since if they exhibited a similar degree of nuclear atypicality and were exophytic, they would qualify for the diagnosis of condyloma acuminatum. A true VIN I lesion without an associated or adjacent higher-grade VIN, usually VIN III, is a relatively unusual finding. In fact, most lesser-grade VIN lesions found in association with VIN III are a minimum of VIN II.

In VIN II lesions, the abnormal cytologic findings extend into the middle to upper two-thirds of the epithelium (Fig. 5.4), and mitotic figures, including more abnormal ones, are easily found. There is some degree of maturation in the upper third of the epithelium.

In VIN III lesions, two-thirds to full thickness of the squamous epithelium is replaced by cells with the cytologic characteristics of cancer; in comparison to the lesser grades of VIN, the cells show a greater population density, greater nuclear pleomorphism, more radial dispersion and coarser clumping of the chromatin, greater wrinkling of the nuclear membrane, increased mitotic activity at all levels of the epithelium, and more abnormal mitotic forms. The "warty" type of VIN III is characterized by an undulating surface configuration often with prominent parakeratosis or hyperkeratosis (Fig. 5.5) and cells showing some degree of maturation and prominent eosinophilic cytoplasm. The "basaloid" type of VIN III is characterized by smaller, more relatively uniform cells (Fig. 5.6) with a more smooth and flat surface.

Although seen in lesser grades of VIN, multinucleated giant cells are more frequent in VIN III. Intracellular and extracellular melanin pigment granules (Fig. 5.7) contribute to those cases of pigmented VIN, and underlying dermal melanophages reflect past pigment incontinence. VIN III extends into the epithelium of the skin appendages (Figs. 5.2, 5.8) in more than half of the cases, and this should not be confused with early invasion.

Despite a benign clinical and gross appearance, lesions once referred to as "BP" can exhibit a paradoxically worrisome microscopic appearance. Some workers have interpreted the latter as equivalent to moderate or severe dysplasia or even as carcinoma in situ, whereas others have acknowledged the striking intraepithelial cellularity and uniformity (Fig. 5.9); they note, however, that there is only a mild degree of cytologic atypia and that any greater degree of atypia is relatively rare (Fig. 5.10). Although mitotic activity is common, abnormal forms of mitotic figures are not typically encountered. Also noted as a frequent finding in "BP" is the absence of hair follicle involvement, although this parameter loses its importance unless the epithelium overlying the follicle is dysplastic. Most workers acknowledge the considerable confusion regarding the microscopic features that characterize "BP", precluding its acceptance as a distinct diagnostically reproducible

histopathologic entity; most workers currently regard it to be a subtype of VIN.

The squamous epithelium affected by POD shows spongiosis accompanied by prominent exocytosis of inflammatory cells. The squamous cells exhibit degenerative changes manifested by swollen, pale-staining and vacuolated cytoplasm and pyknotic nuclei (Fig. 5.11) with dispersed chromatin grains ("podophyllin cells"). Nuclei also may be enlarged and hyperchromatic with nucleoli increased in both size and number. Mitotic figures are present in large numbers, and virtually all are arrested in metaphase of the cell cycle (Fig. 5.12), similar to colchicine-treated epidermis. Particularly in the basal and parabasal layers, there is disintegration of the chromatinic membrane. The findings of disrupted and dispersed chromatin particles as well as chromosomes aggregated in groups of 2 and 3 point toward aborted mitosis as a mechanism whereby topical podophyllin exerts its effect; such can also result in abnormal-appearing mitotic figures that can be confused with the abnormal ones commonly seen with high-grade VIN. However, the foregoing cytoplasmic degenerative changes and the nuclear debris from disruption and dispersal that accompany POD effect are uncommon findings in VIN.

PROGNOSIS AND TREATMENT

The prognosis and treatment for VIN are discussed in Chapter 2. Early reports indicated that many lesions of so-called "BP" would regress spontaneously if untreated; however, the demonstration of the oncogenic HPV type 16 in some cases of "BP" is disturbing. Since many pathologists maintain that "BP" cannot be reliably differentiated from VIN on a histopathologic basis, the ISSVD and the ISGYP have eschewed use of the term. Therefore, since "BP" is regarded as a subset of VIN from a clinical and diagnostic pathology viewpoint, many clinicians treat it as they would any other VIN lesion.

Since the effects of topical POD persist for 2–6 weeks, it should not be applied for a month or two prior to biopsy; further, the pathologist should be informed if the patient was treated with the drug and when it was last used. The histologic effects of POD disappear with time; however, most VIN lesions, particularly the high-grade ones, tend to persist or progress in severity.

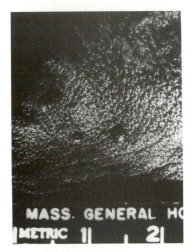

Figure 5.1. Genital skin with papular VIN (clinical diagnosis of "bowenoid papulosis").

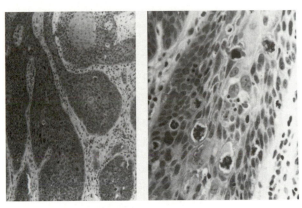

Figure 5.2. VIN III involving adnexal structures.

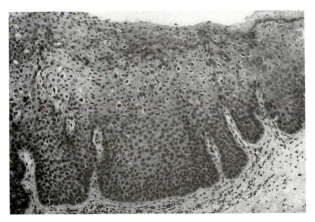

Figure 5.3. VIN I.

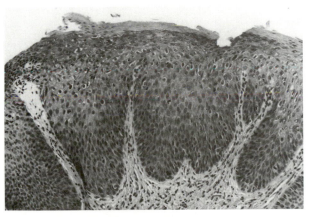

Figure 5.4. VIN II.

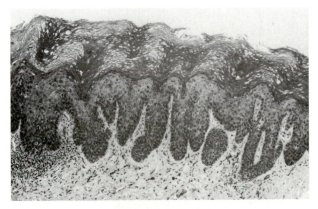

Figure 5.5. VIN III- "warty" type.

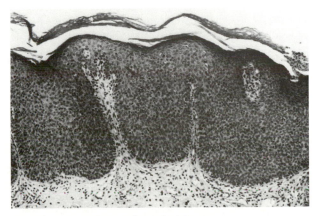

Figure 5.6. VIN III- basaloid type.

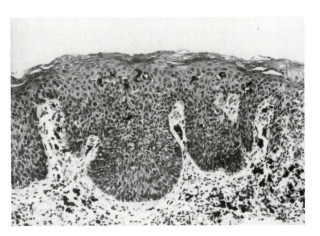

Figure 5.7. VIN III-with numerous intraepithelial pigmented dendritic cells and dermal melanophages.

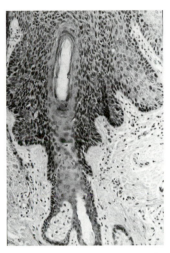

Figure 5.8. VIN III involving hair follicles.

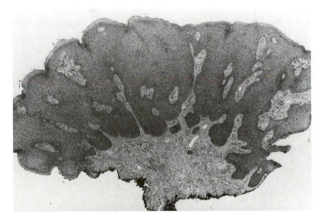

Figure 5.9. Low grade VIN diagnosed clinically as "bowenoid papulosis".

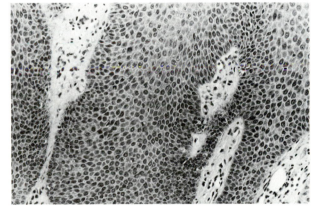

Figure 5.10. Low grade VIN diagnosed clinically as "bowenoid papulosis".

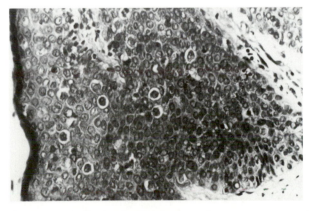

Figure 5.11. Podophyllin-induced squamous atypia.

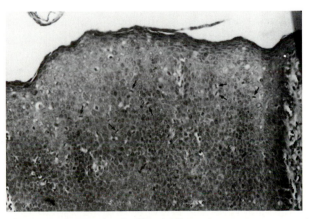

Figure 5.12. Podophyllin-induced squamous atypia. (arrows-mitotic figures arrested in metaphase).

6. Extramammary Paget's Disease

vs.

Pagetoid Spread of Superficial Spreading Melanoma

vs.

"Clear Cell" Change Simulating Paget's Disease

CLINICAL

About two-thirds of patients with extramammary Paget's disease (PD) are older than 60, and almost all are white and postmenopausal. More than half of them complain of longstanding, chronic pruritus, burning, irritation, and general vulvar discomfort. The extent of PD is often roughly proportional to the duration of the symptoms. Any area of the anogenital skin is susceptible to involvement by PD; however, the labia majora are most commonly affected. Because of its protracted and slowly progressive course, PD is often misdiagnosed and treated as an intractable, poorly responsive chronic vulvar dermatitis.

Vulvar melanoma also afflicts predominantly white, postmenopausal women, most of whom are in the 6th to 8th decades. However, approximately a third of them are premenopausal and <50 years of age, findings that are distinctly unusual for PD. Patients complain of bleeding, the presence of a mass, and pruritus. Almost two-thirds of MM arise from either a labium majus or minus or the clitoris. Three distinct histopathologic types of melanoma involve the vulva: nodular melanoma (NM), acral lentiginous melanoma (ALM), and superficial spreading melanoma (SSM); the latter is most likely to be confused with PD because of its propensity for pagetoid spread.

Clear cell change, first described in the skin of the nipple, is an incidental finding in vulvar squamous epithelium and has, to our knowledge, no characteristic clinical findings; however, in patients with a current or prior diagnosis of PD, its presence in either margins of resection for primary resection or in follow-up biopsies for possible recurrence may cause confusion and misdiagnosis.

GROSS

Extramammary PD typically appears as a 1–10-cm-diameter flat or slightly raised erythematous, velvety lesion with scattered white patches; the margins are fairly well demarcated and often irregular in shape. The lesion may have a moist and oozing character with an eczema-tous appearance, contributing to the aforementioned clinical misinterpretation as a longstanding vulvar dermatitis. Ulceration is often a feature, and contact bleeding is common. As previously mentioned, although the labia majora are the most common site, the disease may spread to involve the mons, the thighs, and the lower abdomen. Even the mucosae of the rest of the lower urogenital tract may be involved, including the urethra, bladder, periurethral glands, vagina, and cervix.

SSM typically demonstrates mucosal involvement (Fig. 6.1-arrow), with a labium majus or minus or the clitoris involved in about 75% of cases. Most of them are 0.5–10 cm in diameter (mean 2.5 cm) at the time of detection, and two thirds are pigmented in varying degrees and shades of brown, black, blue, and gray. Some are poorly to nonpigmented (amelanotic).

Clear cell change of the vulvar squamous epithelium has no associated typical gross characteristics.

HISTOPATHOLOGY

PD is currently regarded by the International Society for the Study of Vulvar Disease and the International Society of Gynecological Pathologists as a subcategory of VIN, representing an in situ adenocarcinoma within an otherwise relatively normal-appearing vulvar squamous epithelium; such intraepithelial adenocarcinoma cells may originate primarily in the epidermis, or they may arise in an underlying adenocarcinoma and migrate upward to infiltrate the squamous epithelium. Less commonly, there may be intraepithelial pagetoid extension to vulvar squamous epithelium from an otherwise typical primary carcinoma of the rectum, cervix, endometrium, or bladder.

Paget's cells are large, polygonal cells (Fig. 6.2) with abundant amphophilic to basophilic or clear cytoplasm scattered singly or in small groups among the keratinocytes (Fig. 6.3); predominantly the basal and parabasal layers of the squamous epithelium and the pilosebaceous apparatus (Fig. 6.4) are involved. Occasionally, gland-like acini (Fig. 6.5) are formed, as are signet-ring forms (Fig. 6.3). Nuclei may vary in their degree of atypicality; in some cases the chromatin is open and vesicular and in others more coarsely clumped. Nucleoli are prominent but not markedly enlarged. Mitotic figures are seldom a prominent feature. The Paget's cells spread laterally throughout the squamous epithelium and at the outer limits of the lesion may be present in relatively sparse numbers.

Special stains for neutral and acid mucins, including PAS, Alcian blue, and mucicarmine (Fig. 6.6), show intracytoplasmic positivity. Immunohistochemical stains that are positive in PD include CEA (Fig. 6.7), epithelial membrane antigen, gross cystic disease fluid protein-15, and some, but not all, keratins. Furthermore, Paget's cells have a well-recognized capacity to invade the dermis (Fig. 6.8—arrows) as an invasive adenocarcinoma.

NM shows no radial growth phase with pagetoid spread. ALM, often encountered in the vestibule and characterized by spindly melanocytes extending into the dermis in a diffuse pattern, typically exhibits little to no pagetoid spread. The malignant melanocytes within an invasive focus of SSM are often large with uniform nuclei and prominent nucleoli. Cells with similar characteristics may infiltrate the adjacent epithelium as the "radial growth phase" (by definition, involving 4 or more adjacent rete ridges). The abundant epithelioid malignant melanocytes, sometimes with clear cytoplasm, that are scattered throughout the epithelium also assume a pagetoid pattern (Fig. 6.9), further heightening the resemblance to PD.

Special stains for the aforementioned mucins are always negative in melanoma. Melanin stains are of no differential utility because Paget's cells sometimes engulf melanin, as is shown by the arrow in Fig. 6.10, or the malignant melanocytes may be largely amelanotic (Fig. 6.11), closely resembling the Paget's cells depicted in Figure 6.10. Immunohistochemical stains show negativity in melanoma for cytokeratins and the usual positivity for HMB-45 and S-100; PD is negative for the latter two.

Clear cell change has been described in the skin of the nipple as an incidental finding but may also be seen in vulvar skin. The cells appear to be keratinocytes with small hyperchromatic nuclei and clear cytoplasm (Fig. 6.12); the latter is likely due to hydropic change since special stains for intracytoplasmic glycogen and mucin are negative. The cytologic changes are not those of HPV effect.

PROGNOSIS AND TREATMENT

The prognosis for noninvasive PD is excellent, and the primary treatment consists of wide excision of the involved area down to the fascia. Adequate margins of normal tissue are desirable, and frozen-section diagnosis may be used to assist in their evaluation. However, Paget's cells have a well-known propensity to exist in small numbers in the grossly and histologically normal-appearing skin of resection margins. Indeed, they may be present and easily overlooked. Conversely, the section submitted for frozen-section diagnosis may show no Paget's cells, and the next deeper cut in the paraffin block taken for permanent section may contain sparse numbers of them. Consequently, although it is helpful, frozen-section diagnosis is not absolutely reliable in establishing the status of the resection margins in PD. The finding of a few Paget's cells in normal-appearing skin adjacent to overt PD explains many ostensibly recurrent cases; in actuality, the latter probably represent persistent disease, which is also treated successfully by local excision.

Early detection and diagnosis of vulvar melanoma is the mainstay of treatment; therefore, an adequate skin examination of the vulva is mandatory. The depth of invasion is the single most important factor in determining the subsequent biologic behavior of melanomas; indeed, early, minimally invasive SSMs have a significantly better prognosis and longer survival than do more deeply invasive ones. Good prognostic parameters include a thickness of ≤0.75 mm, 1.49 mm in overall thickness, and a Clark level II or less. Adverse prognostic parameters are found more frequently in larger tumors and include an overall thickness of >2 mm or a Clark level V, mitotic count of >10/mm^2, vascular space invasion, tumor necrosis, a sparse or absent inflammatory response in the dermis, and surface ulceration of the lesion.

Clear cell change in the epidermis has no known effect on prognosis or treatment except for the potential sequelae of its misdiagnosis as either a false-positive margin or recurrence in a patient with primary PD or a history of treated PD.

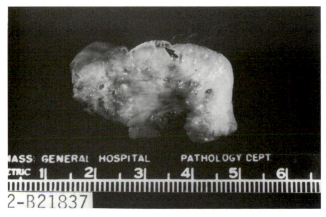

Figure 6.1. Superficially spreading vulvar malignant melanoma (arrow).

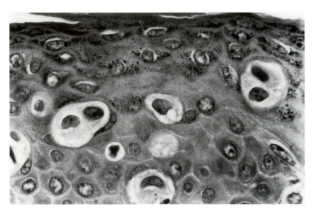

Figure 6.2. Vulvar Paget's disease.

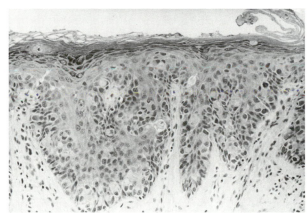

Figure 6.3. Vulvar Paget's disease.

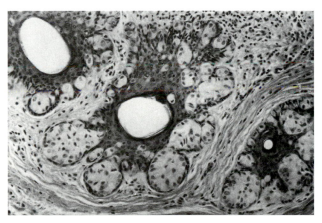

Figure 6.4. Vulvar Paget's disease involving adnexac.

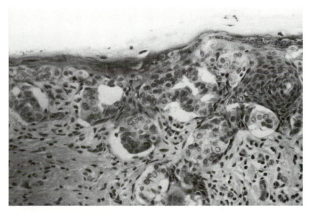

Figure 6.5. Vulvar Paget's disease exhibiting gland formation.

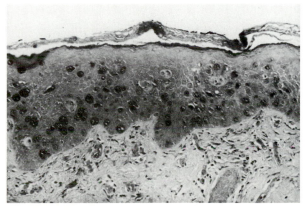

Figure 6.6. Vulvar Paget's disease (mucicarmine stain).

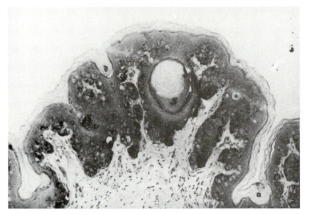

Figure 6.7. Vulvar Paget's disease (immunostain for carcinoembryonic antigen).

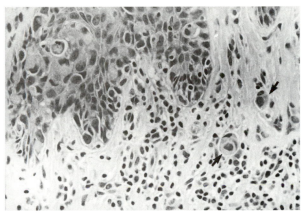

Figure 6.8. Vulvar Paget's disease with superficial dermal invasion (arrows).

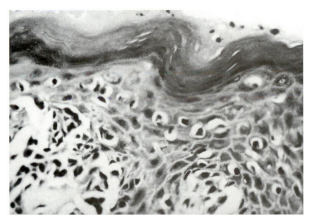

Figure 6.9. Superficial spreading vulvar malignant melanoma with pagetoid pattern of spread.

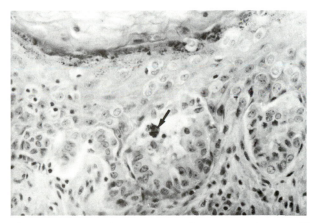

Figure 6.10. Vulvar Paget's disease with engulfed melanin in Paget's cells (arrow).

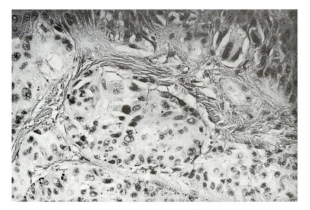

Figure 6.11. Superficial spreading vulvar malignant melanoma, largely amelanotic.

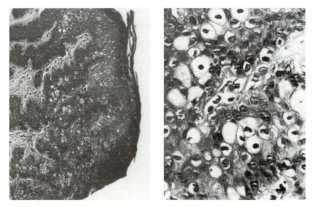

Figure 6.12. "Clear cells" within vulvar epidermis, mimicking Paget's disease.

7. Atypical Nevomelanocytic Nevi of Genital Type in Young Premenopausal Women

vs.

Mucocutaneous Superficial Spreading Malignant Melanoma

CLINICAL

Atypical nevomelanocytic nevi (ANN) may represent a relatively infrequently encountered, but probably distinctive, form of nevus on the vulva or perineum in premenopausal females between 20 and 30 years old. ANN are usually asymptomatic and discovered during a routine gynecologic examination. About a third of them may be discovered during pregnancy or in patients taking oral contraceptives. ANN are not uncommonly encountered in consultation practice, where they are sent with the query "rule out malignant melanoma arising in association with a dermal nevus."

The clinicopathologic types of malignant melanoma (MM) are mentioned in Chapter 6. The SSM and ALM types, particularly in their so-called radial growth phase, are more likely to be confused with atypical nevomelanocytic lesions. A malignant melanoma in radial growth phase typically appears as a pigmented plaque that has been growing slowly by circumferential enlargement over a period of months to years. Its contour is often markedly irregular, and the surface appears variegated in color. Some areas may be intensely brown-black, whereas others may display hypopigmentation, sometimes representing regressing melanoma.

GROSS

The ANN of adolescent girls and young premenopausal women are small, with a mean diameter of 5–6 mm, and their borders are fairly well circumscribed (Fig. 7.1). Often elevated or polypoid, the ANN usually has a tan to brown coloration, although a third or so of them may display some black pigmentation. MM often display variegated pigmentation, a worrisome finding when attempting to differentiate between MM and benign or atypical pigmented lesions. MM may be flat, ulcerated, nodular, or polypoid. Various shades of pigmentation may be present in the skin or mucosa adjacent to the tumor, as may so-called satellite nodules of MM.

HISTOPATHOLOGY

The histopathologic appearance of ANN in young premenopausal females is typified by a distinctive and symmetrical type of melanocytic nesting, composed of epithelioid and spindled nevus cells, in the epidermis and at the dermal–epidermal interface (Fig. 7.2). Indeed, at the latter there is a characteristic crowding of the nests and lesional melanocytes, thereby encroaching on and obscuring the undersurface of the basal aspect of the epidermis and making difficult the identification of individual nests entirely within the epidermis (Fig. 7.2). Atypical but benign pagetoid cells similar to those seen in the characteristic intraepidermal and dermal nests may also be encountered within ANN. This is not a particularly worrisome finding as long as they remain cytologically bland. In ANN, extension of the aforementioned atypical melanocytic nests into the dermis, especially in florid examples (Figs. 7.2, 7.3), may lead to the erroneous diagnosis of invasive MM; however, in ANN there is definite maturation of the cells infiltrating the deeper dermis (Fig. 7.4). The lymphoid infiltrate is often scattered and inconspicuous in ANN.

The radial growth phase of SSMs and ALMs is characterized by variable hyperplasia of markedly atypical melanocytes; the latter diffusely infiltrate the squamous epithelium, often in a pagetoid pattern (Fig. 7.5). Compared to that of SSM, the radial growth phase of ALM more often may show spindled or dendritic atypical melanocytes, more prominent hyperplasia of the rete ridges, and deep involvement of eccrine glands. Both SSM and ALM may exhibit superficial stromal invasion of either the papillary dermis or the superficial vascular plexus. In the radial growth phase, the papillary dermis is invaded by pleomorphic melanocytes (Fig. 7.6), nests of which often appear similar in size to those both within the epidermis and at the dermal–epidermal junction. In contrast, melanocytic nests within a superficial spreading melanoma may be located within and at different levels of the epidermis. Pagetoid extension of malignant melanocytic cells into the epidermis is common in SSM (Fig. 7.6). In MM, many nests, often morphologically heterogeneous (Fig. 7.5), are present within the dermis, and maturation is exceptional.

PROGNOSIS AND TREATMENT

The ANN of young and premenopausal women apparently has little to no risk for developing into MM. Because of its worrisome histologic appearance, it is imperative that ANN not be confused with MM and result in overtreatment.

Although very few vulvar nevi develop into MM, about one-third of vulvar MM arise in preexisting nevi. During examination of the external genitalia, all anogenital nevi occurring on both the skin and mucous membranes should be objectively assessed and carefully described, using written notation of their location, size, color, and any other distinguishing characteristics. Excisional biopsy, taken at a sufficient depth to assure adequacy of dermal encompassment, may be diagnostic and curative. The prognosis and treatment aspects of MM are discussed in Chapter 6.

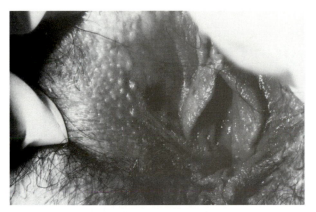

Figure 7.1. Atypical nevomelanocytic nevus-vulva of young female.

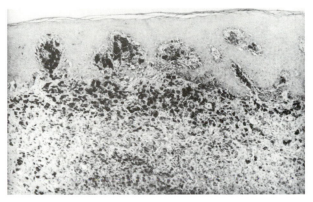

Figure 7.2. Atypical nevomelanocytic nevus-vulva of young female.

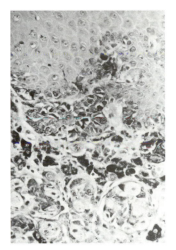

Figure 7.3. Atypical nevomelanocytic nevus-vulva of young female.

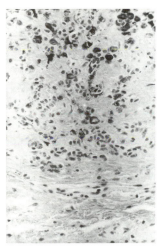

Figure 7.4. Atypical nevomelanocytic nevus-vulva of young female. Note cytologic maturation with increasing depth of the lesion.

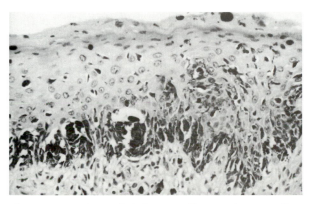

Figure 7.5. Superficial spreading vulvar malignant melanoma.

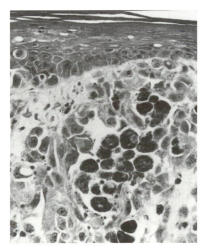

Figure 7.6. Vulvar malignant melanoma.

8. Vulvar Vestibular Papillomas (Papillomatosis)

vs.

Fibroepithelial Squamous Polyp (Achrocordon)

vs.

Condyloma Acuminatum

CLINICAL

The differential diagnosis of the following proliferative squamous lesions that occur in the lower female genital tract is important to preclude the misdiagnosis of a non-venereal disease as a sexually transmitted one with its consequent social ramifications, inherently precancerous potential, and therapeutic implications.

Although vulvar squamous papillomas may occur as a benign, solitary, tumor occurring in middle-aged and older women, they may be confined to the vulvar vestibule, where they typically cluster as multiple papillomas, a finding that has prompted the term *vestibular papillomatosis* (VP). Some regard VP lesions as normal anatomic variations, designating them as "vulvar vestibular papillae," due to their symmetrical distribution and their frequency in completely asymptomatic women. VPs may be associated with pruritus, a burning sensation, or dyspareunia. The fibroepithelial squamous polyp (FEP), or achrocordon, is usually solitary and arises only from the hairbearing skin of the vulva. Condyloma acuminata (CDLA) typically occur in young, sexually active women, and multiple anogenital sites may be affected.

GROSS

VPs appear on the lateral vestibular mucosal surfaces as tiny, soft, and pliable papillae or exhibit a roughened, "pebble grain" appearance. CDLAs display multiple spikes from a common stalk and are covered by a thick layer of white epithelium, but each of the papillae in VP arises independently from the surface mucosa and varies in length from 1 to 5 mm. FEPs are usually soft, and commonly pedunculated (Fig. 8.1) with a finely lobulated or wrinkled ("mulberry" type) surface that is usually the color of the skin from which they arise, although the tip may be hypopigmented. In the rare case where they are multiple, clustering is not a feature.

Three-quarters of CDLA begin as small, pale gray to white, sessile growths or lesions with a central stalk and multiple complex finger-like projections. CDLA expand by coalescence to form confluent masses. Exophytic lobulated tumors are more typical of older lesions; however, untreated advanced lesions may paradoxically flatten as they spread to involve large areas of the anogenital area.

HISTOPATHOLOGY

The papillae of VPs are covered by a thin squamous epithelium with minimal to no hyperkeratosis; although clustered, the villi are isolated and separate (Fig. 8.2), possessing a central vascular core without the branching and arborizing typical of CDLA. Cytologic features similar to those seen with HPV-related changes are rarely observed, (Fig. 8.3) or are subtle and restricted to the bases of the fronds. Newer molecular biologic techniques have indicated the presence of HPV DNA in a minority of lesions otherwise typical of VP. The FEP shows no villous or papillary architecture (Fig. 8.4) but displays, on the other hand, the configuration of a single polyp, often with a stalk. Its squamous lining also exhibits some acanthosis and hyperkeratosis but typically is thinner than that of the VP. Importantly, the squamous epithelium of neither the VP nor the FEP exhibits clearcut evidence of HPV infection. The squamous epithelium of CDLA shows an exuberant squamous cell hyperplasia superimposed on delicate, branching, and arborizing fibrovascular cores (Fig. 8.5); also there is papillomatosis, acanthosis with prominent desmosomes, elongated and narrow rete pegs, and marked hyperkeratosis. Koilocytes are prominent (Fig. 8.6), especially in the superficial squamous layers. Binucleation and multinucleation may occur, but significant nuclear atypia is seldom seen.

PROGNOSIS AND TREATMENT

For symptomatic VPs, local ablative or topical measures are effective. Those who consider VPs as a normal genital variant caution against their misdiagnosis and treatment as HPV-related lesions, particularly when asymptomatic; however, the demonstration of HPV DNA in a small number of VPs is supportive of probable venereal transmission in at least a minority of them. FEPs are easily treated with simple surgical excision. A plethora of treatment modalities have been attempted for CDLA, including cytotoxic agents such as podophyllin, 5FU (5-Fluorouracil) trichloroacetic acid, interferon, cryosurgery, laser ablation, and most currently, loop-excision electrocautery procedures (LEEP).

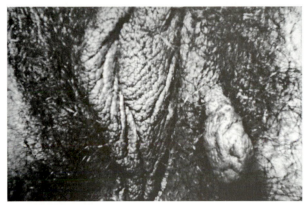

Figure 8.1. Vulvar fibroepithelial polyp.

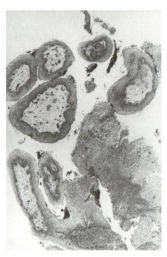

Figure 8.2. Vulvar vestibular papillomatosis.

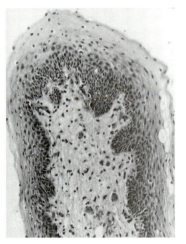

Figure 8.3. Vulvar vestibular papillomatosis.

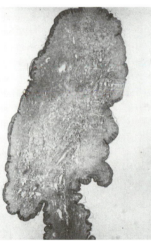

Figure 8.4. Vulvar fibroepithelial polyp.

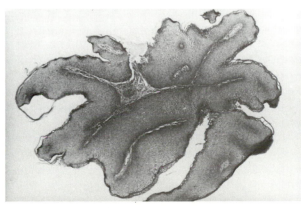

Figure 8.5. Vulvar condyloma acuminatum.

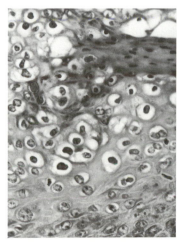

Figure 8.6. Vulvar condyloma acuminatum with prominent koilocytes.

9. Keratoacanthoma

vs.

Verrucous Carcinoma

vs.

Warty (Condylomatous) Squamous Carcinoma

CLINICAL

About 10% of keratoacanthomas (KAs) occur in nonexposed skin, and infrequently involve the hairbearing portions of the vulva in older women. Vulvar KA are self-limiting and noted for rapid growth for 6–8 weeks, followed by apparent nongrowth and then eventual regression over ~6 months.

Verrucous carcinoma (VC) is a rare and apparently distinct form of very well-differentiated squamous cell carcinoma (SCC). The mean age is in the 7th decade, and VC is distinctly uncommon in premenopausal women. In one large series half the patients had a history of biopsy-proven condyloma (CDLA) 3–10 years prior to diagnosis; indeed, for many years VC was known as the giant condyloma of Buschke and Lowenstein.

VCs are slow-growing, warty vulvar lesions often present for years; consequently, most are quite large by the time of initial diagnosis. VCs have been mistakenly treated as refractory condyloma; however, the considerably older age of patients with VC, compared to those with typical CDLA, should arouse the suspicion of malignancy.

The clinical characteristics in general of vulvar SCCs are discussed in Chapter 4. The histopathologic subtype of SCC most likely to be confused with VC is the warty or condylomatous variety. Warty SCCs often harbor HPV, particularly the oncogenic serotype 16, and they generally occur in younger women. In one study, a history of antecedent malignancy in the lower genital tract, including the cervix and other vulvar sites, was common. One-third of them were multifocal.

GROSS

Vulvar KA typically is a solitary, firm, raised nodule that measures between 1 and 2.5 cm in diameter, although most never surpass 4 or 5 cm in diameter. The surface is dome-shaped and irregular, and the center is occupied by a horn-filled crater; a "warty" surface configuration is not characteristic of KA.

VCs may closely resemble CDLA. Small VCs have been reported so that early forms may overlap on a size basis with both KAs and smaller SCCs. The typical VC arises on a labium majus as a large, fungating, cauliflower-like mass ≥10 cm in diameter, frequently described as "warty" on gross examination. On cut section, the tumor–stromal junction is sharp and well demarcated, exhibiting a smooth, scalloped pushing border (Fig. 9.1), rather than a ragged and irregularly infiltrating one.

The warty type of SCC, like VC, is often a large, exophytic tumor with a nodular or papillary configuration (a "verruciform" appearance). On cut section, however, the tumor–stromal interface of the warty SCC is irregular, ragged, and poorly delineated.

HISTOPATHOLOGY

An adequate biopsy, preferably of the entire lesion to include the deep and lateral borders, is important in the microscopic evaluation of a KA since its architectural features are as important as the cytologic ones. The prototypical KA has a paradoxical histopathologic appearance, composed of a benign-appearing, well-differentiated squamous epithelium with glassy eosinophilic cytoplasm (Fig. 9.2) surrounding a central crater filled with keratin; however, the lateral and deep aspects of the lesion are marked by irregular, infiltrative-appearing borders (Fig. 9.3). Such an appearance is easily confused with superficially invasive SCC both at low magnification (Fig. 9.4) and on higher-power examination (Fig. 9.5). The borders of KAs are generally better defined than in invasive SCCs, and KAs usually exhibit a greater degree of overall symmetry than SCC. The central keratin-filled crater is not a prominent feature in most invasive SCCs.

Actually, KAs are less atypical appearing in the fully developed stage than in the early, proliferative stage, where there may be considerable nuclear atypia and even perineural invasion. The epidermis at the margin of the lesion extends as a "lip," designated by the arrow in Figure 9.6, over the sides of the central keratin-filled crater. However, squamous carcinomas certainly may show a similar phenomenon, exemplified by the squamous carcinoma illustrated in Figure 9.7, further heightening the possibility of confusion between the two entities. The base of a KA, despite the resemblance of individual small nests to SCC, is relatively regular at low magnification and seldom extends below the level of the sweat glands. The healing or involuted stage of KA is less apt to be confused with SCC. In involuted KAs there is a greater degree of keratinization observed in the cup-like base of the lesion. There is usually a dense lichenoid type of inflammatory infiltrate at the interface with the stroma. Eosinophils may be a prominent component of the infiltrate, providing a helpful differential point against SCC since the latter seldom exhibits such. In contrast, plasma cells frequently are present in large numbers in the inflammatory infiltrate bordering invasive SCCs, an unusual finding in KA.

The surface of VC is composed of exophytic papillary fronds (Fig. 9.8). Hyperkeratosis and parakeratosis are variable but usually extensive. Although the surface architectural features are reminiscent of CDLA, the characteristic central fibrovascular stalks of condyloma are absent. The rete ridges are composed of well-differentiated squamous cells containing abundant eosinophilic cytoplasm; clearcut cytologic features of malignancy are absent. Squamous pearl formation is not a frequent feature. Nuclear atypia may occur focally in the bases of the rete pegs, but nuclei are generally bland and uniform, exhibiting only mild pleomorphism (Fig. 9.9). Mitotic activity is rare. When present, mitoses are confined to the basal and parabasal strata; most mitotic figures are typical but occasionally abnormal forms will be identified.

In the deeper portion of the epithelium in VCs, there is extensive and striking acanthosis associated with bulbous enlargement of the rete pegs (Fig. 9.10); the latter extend below the level of the surrounding normal epidermis and represent a largely endophytic, or "pushing," type of invasion rather than a destructive, aggressive manner of infiltration. The tumor–stromal interface is well delimited, and a chronic inflammatory infiltrate is often present in the dermis. It is imperative to remember that any vulvar SCC with the above-mentioned architectural features, regardless of the histopathologic subtype, does not belong in the category of VC unless the criteria of bland and innocuous cytologic features, with minimal nuclear atypia, are present within a very highly differentiated SCC.

Warty SCC has a papillary well-differentiated surface that is often thrown into spikes that contain fibrovascular cores reminiscent of CDLA. Cytologic changes due to HPV effect are common and are especially evident in the overlying warty VIN. Papilloma virus-like particles have been identified within two-thirds of warty SCCs by ultrastructural studies. However, nuclear atypicality certainly is greater than that seen with typical CDLA or even VC, and intraepithelial squamous pearls may be seen. The majority of warty SCCs are superficially invasive, and relatively few invade to a depth of 4 mm. In contrast to the VC, the basal aspect of the tumor is jagged and irregular and the tumor–stromal interface is ragged (Fig. 9.11). Small, irregularly shaped nests and cords of tumor invade the dermis (Fig. 9.12).

PROGNOSIS AND TREATMENT

Most KAs regress and involute within ~6 months to a flattened fibrous scar. When the distinction between KA and SCC is difficult, a more prudent course may be to treat the lesion as an invasive SCC; an explanatory note stating that a KA cannot be excluded unequivocally may be appended. However, every effort should be made to differentiate the two since the diagnosis of invasive SCC may be followed by radical surgery.

VC is generally a slow-growing tumor that is known for locally aggressive behavior, often invading surrounding anogenital soft tissues and bone. Extranodal or nodal metastases should at least raise suspicion about the correctness of the original diagnosis of VC. Currently, most VC are treated by either complete excision of the lesion with wide margins (at least 2 cm of surrounding normal tissue), or total vulvectomy with lymphadenectomy (particularly in very large lesions). The 5-year survival of completely excised VC is close to 95% and death, which occurs in only a small minority of patients, is usually from consequences of extensive and massive local recurrence.

Some workers have suggested that ionizing radiation transforms otherwise typical VC in as many as 10% of patients, to a much higher-grade tumor or even anaplastic SCC (some within a period of 2 months after receiving radiation therapy); however, the role of radiation in the biologic behavior of VC is still considered controversial at present.

The prognosis of warty SCC has been suggested to lie somewhere between VC and conventional SCC. Wide local excision or total vulvectomy may be adequate treatment.

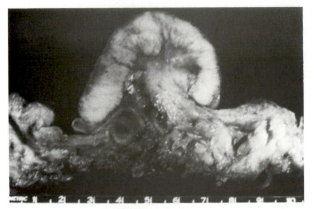

Figure 9.1. Verrucous carcinoma of vulva.

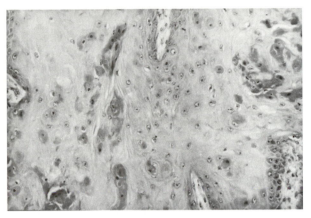

Figure 9.2. Vulvar keratoacanthoma.

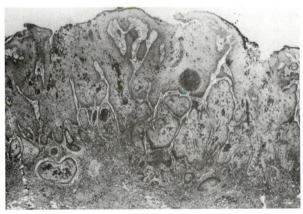

Figure 9.3. Vulvar keratoacanthoma.

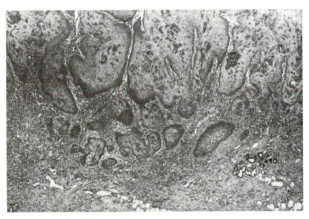

Figure 9.4. Vulvar keratoacanthoma.

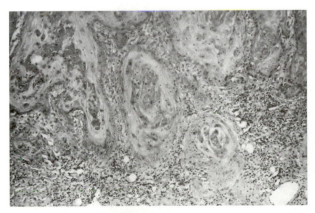

Figure 9.5. Vulvar keratoacanthoma.

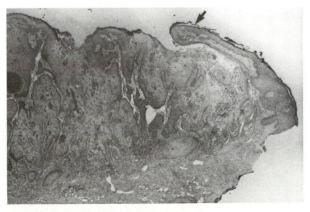

Figure 9.6. Vulvar keratoacanthoma.

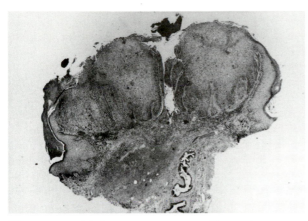

Figure 9.7. Vulvar squamous cell carcinoma.

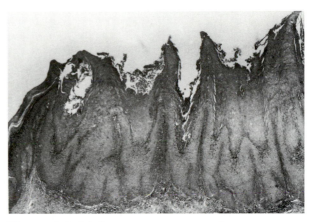

Figure 9.8. Vulvar verrucous carcinoma.

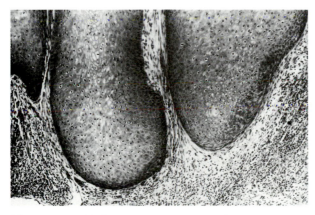

Figure 9.9. Vulvar verrucous carcinoma.

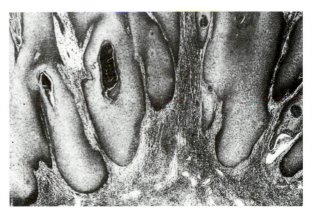

Figure 9.10. Vulvar verrucous carcinoma.

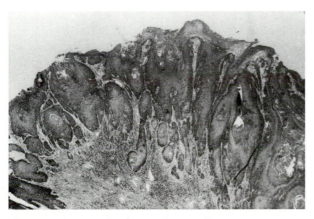

Figure 9.11. Vulvar "warty" squamous cell carcinoma.

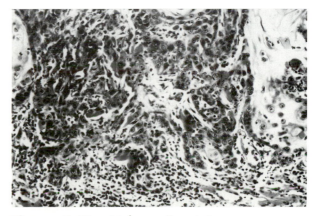

Figure 9.12. Vulvar "warty" squamous cell carcinoma.

10. Basal Cell Carcinoma with Adenoid Pattern (Adenoid Basal Cell Carcinoma)

vs.

Adenoid Cystic Carcinoma (Bartholin Gland) vs. Basaloid (Squamous) Carcinoma of Anal Canal Involving Anogenital Area

CLINICAL

The most important differential diagnostic point to be made among these three entities is that the relatively low-grade basal cell carcinoma (BCC) with adenoid pattern should not be confused with the other two highly malignant tumors. Although typical vulvar BCC is uncommon (3–13% of all vulvar malignancies), the subtype of BCC with adenoid pattern is even less common. BCC typically occurs in skin exposed to actinic radiation, but it may be caused by other conditions, including x-rays and arsenical compounds. BCC are usually encountered in middle-aged or elderly white postmenopausal women. Three-quarters of anogenital BCCs arise on the labia majora, particularly the anterior portions; however, they can arise in areas favored by adenoid cystic carcinomas. The BCC with adenoid pattern has no clinical characteristics to separate it from the typical BCC.

Adenoid cystic carcinoma (ACC) is also a rare vulvar cancer, occurring with similar frequency as BCC (reported incidence range 3–8%). Most ACCs occur in perimenopausal or postmenopausal women in the 6th decade. The tumor often presents as a palpable, tender, and indurated mass with or without ulceration. Although often mistaken clinically for a benign inflammatory or cystic lesion, particularly a Bartholin cyst, this is a dangerous assumption in women over 40 years old, an age group in which inflammatory phenomena are less common and neoplastic ones more likely.

The so-called basaloid type of squamous carcinoma (BSC), which may arise from the anal canal and spread upward to involve the genital and perigenital skin, should be differentiated from BCC and ACC. Although BSC is the least commonly encountered cancer of the anal canal, it is twice as frequent in women; furthermore, female patients with BSC have an increased incidence of lower genital tract carcinomas, especially of the cervix. BSC usually presents little problem in clinical or patho-logic diagnosis. However, occasionally some of them exhibit features that cause confusion with either BCC or ACC. A careful history and clinical examination should suggest the primary source of the tumor.

GROSS

An ulcerated, raised, or nodular mass is the most common presentation in vulvar BCC; however, BCC may present as a cystic or papillary lesion. Other less common gross manifestations include an erythematous plaque, a white patch, or even a hyperpigmented dark brown to black lesion that may be confused with malignant melanoma. Most BCCs are ≤2 cm in diameter, although in rare cases ≥10-cm BCCs have been described. They are generally firm and have well-defined borders; the appearance of sharply defined "rolled edges" is often, but by no means invariably, present.

Particularly in those smaller-diameter ACCs, which have yet to distort the vulvar anatomy, ACC typically arises from the site of a Bartholin gland and has a predilection for the left side. It may vary in size from 1 to ≥7 cm in diameter. Although frequently cystic on cut section, a solid component often imparts, even on gross examination, the appearance of an aggressive tumor with deep invasion into the underlying tissues. Such a gross picture would be a distinctly unusual finding in BCC.

BSC of the anal canal, particularly if it has spread extensively to involve the genital and perigenital tissues, has a likewise aggressive appearance. BSC exhibits nonspecific tumor necrosis and friability.

HISTOPATHOLOGY

The histopathologic patterns of typical vulvar BCC appear similar to those arising in extragenital epidermis.

Most commonly, solid nests and islands of uniform cells arise from the basal aspect of the epidermis and superficially invade the dermis (Fig. 10.1). The predominant cell type is small, monotonous, and basaloid with sparse cytoplasm and a small, dense hyperchromatic nucleus. However, some BCCs exhibit more nuclear pleomorphism and a higher mitotic index. Cystic degeneration and necrosis may impart a more worrisome appearance to the tumor. The degree of mitotic activity is variable but is rarely particularly brisk. Characteristic changes of the connective-tissue stroma also may be prominent, including hyalinization or a myxoid or mucoid appearance. A rather characteristic "crack artifact" is often seen around the invading nests of tumor.

The subtype of BCC referred to as BCC with adenoid pattern is characterized by a focal but notable microacinar and cribriform glandular component that is readily apparent, even on low-power examination (Fig. 10.2). BCCs with adenoid pattern often arise from the basal layer of the epidermis and grow in a serpentine manner. The cribriform glandular patterns (Fig. 10.3) may be accompanied by tubular formations (Fig. 10.4); the latter may be intimately associated with more solid areas of BCC as well as by evidence of squamous differentiation. Peripheral palisading is a frequent feature. Use of the term *BCC with adenoid pattern* is preferable to *adenoid BCC*. This avoids confusion with the cervical tumor known as *adenoid basal carcinoma* (ABC), which has a microscopic appearance different from that of the BCC-with-adenoid pattern. To confuse them could imply a metastasis to the vulva from a cervical tumor that has never shown convincing evidence of metastasis. Likewise, the designation of BCC with adenoid cystic pattern or adenocystic BCC should be discouraged because of the obvious risk of confusion with ACC.

Vulvar ACC has a microscopic appearance, even on low-power examination (Fig. 10.5), which is similar to ACCs described in extragenital sites such as the breast and salivary glands. Uniform basaloid cells constitute nests, islands, and cords in which are interspersed variable-sized microglandular structures (Figs. 10.6, 10.7). The microcysts generally contain either a mucinous or an eosinophilic basement membrane–like material; the latter, when viewed in longitudinal section, imparts a tubular or cylindromatous appearance. The stroma may exhibit focal hyalinization (Fig. 10.6). The small glandular structures are lined by a double layer of malignant epithelial and myoepithelial cells, accounting for the positive staining with both cytokeratin and S-100 (Fig. 10.8) in ACC. Perineural invasion is a frequent finding.

Some workers regard BSC of the anus to be essentially a squamous cell carcinoma that may show divergent glandular differentiation. Such tumors may display mixtures of squamous and mucinous cells, the latter in the form of microcystic glands reminiscent of the mucoepidermoid carcinoma of salivary derivation. BSC may present the picture of a high-grade spindled cell carcinoma replacing the mucosa as an intraepithelial component (Figs. 10.9, 10.10) and extending into the submucosa, with extensive vascular space invasion (Fig. 10.10—arrows). BSC frequently contain foci that resemble BCC of the skin and rarely large areas, or even an entire tumor, may be composed of such patterns. Indeed, tumor nests may consist of high-grade spindled squamoid areas that merge with small, largely uniform, and basaloid cells (Figs. 10.11, 10.12) attempting to palisade at the periphery; small gland-like structures reminiscent of those in the aforementioned ACC and BCC with adenoid pattern may be present (Figs. 10.11, 10.12). Like ACC, tumor necrosis is usually extensive and mitotic activity is high, in contrast to BCC with adenoid pattern. Evidence of extensive and widespread invasion is likewise in contradistinction to BCC.

PROGNOSIS AND TREATMENT

Typically, vulvar BCC exhibits locally invasive growth so that its prognosis is excellent and no different from BCC arising from other primary sites. After wide local excision with adequate margins (the most commonly recommended treatment), up to 20% of patients experience recurrent, but easily treatable, tumor. To our knowledge no deaths have ever been reported from vulvar BCC.

Vulvar ACC has a relatively poor prognosis, often because of its confusion with a benign lesion of the Bartholin gland and delay in treatment. However, patient survival with ACC still is purported to be better than with the more common squamous cell carcinoma or usual adenocarcinoma of Bartholin's gland. ACC is typically an insidious tumor marked by slow, relentless growth with a tendency for local recurrence. Distant metastasis tends to occur later in the course of the disease, particularly after local recurrences.

To avoid misdiagnosis as a benign lesion, biopsy of deep tissues in the Bartholin gland area is advisable. All Bartholin gland tissue, particularly from women >40 years of age, should be processed and examined carefully for the presence of concomitant tumor. Although the previous treatment for vulvar ACC was radical vulvectomy with bilateral inguinal–femoral lymph node dissection, some current workers favor wide local excision of the tumor with an ipsilateral inguinal–femoral lymph node dissection.

The prognosis of basaloid carcinoma of the anal canal is closely related to stage and degree of differentiation.

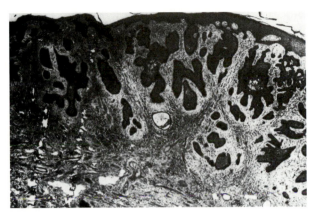

Figure 10.1. Vulvar basal cell carcinoma-usual type.

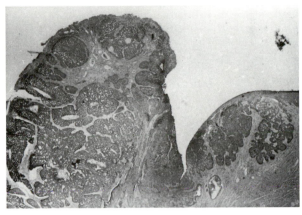

Figure 10.2. Vulvar basal cell carcinoma with adenoid pattern.

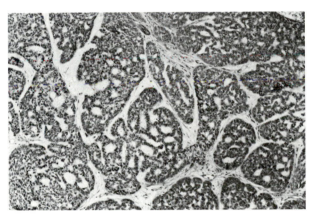

Figure 10.3. Vulvar basal cell carcinoma with adenoid pattern.

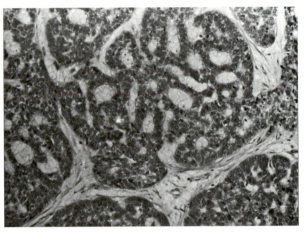

Figure 10.4. Vulvar basal cell carcinoma with adenoid pattern.

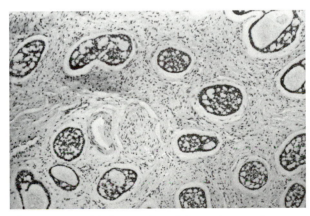

Figure 10.5. Vulvar adenoid cystic carcinoma.

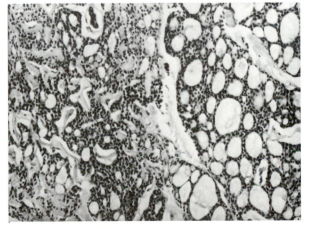

Figure 10.6. Vulvar adenoid cystic carcinoma.

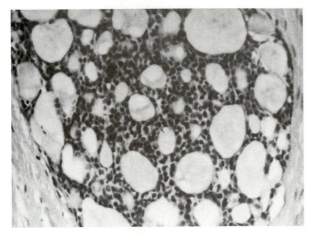

Figure 10.7. Vulvar adenoid cystic carcinoma.

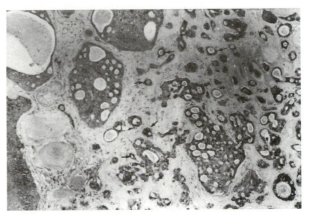

Figure 10.8. Vulvar adenoid cystic carcinoma (immunostain for S-100; arrows).

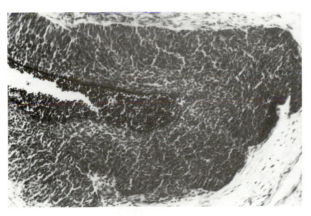

Figure 10.9. Anogenital basaloid squamous carcinoma.

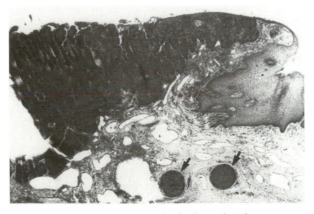

Figure 10.10. Anogenital basaloid squamous carcinoma.

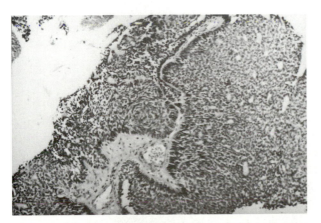

Figure 10.11. Anogenital basaloid squamous carcinoma with small gland-like structures.

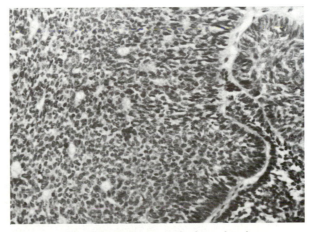

Figure 10.12. Anogenital basaloid squamous carcinoma with small gland-like structures.

11. Bartholin Cyst

vs.

Mucus Cyst of the Vulvar Vestibule

vs.

Mesonephric Cyst

vs.

Mesothelial Cyst of Canal of Nuck

CLINICAL

Vulvar cysts are relatively common, and Bartholin cysts (BCs), which usually arise in reproductive-age women from the paired Bartholin (major vestibular) glands between the urethral meatus and the fourchette, are the most frequent. Most are unilateral, small, and asymptomatic. Their differential diagnosis includes large epidermal cysts, hydroceles and hernias, benign soft tissue tumors such as lipomas and fibromas, and accessory breast tissue.

Mucus cysts of the vulvar vestibule (MCVV) are uncommon, and most are nontender and asymptomatic. Some refer to them as "dysontogenetic" cysts since they likely arise not from mullerian remnants but from obstruction of the ducts of the vulvar minor vestibular glands (urogenital sinus). MCVVs affect mainly parous women or women with a history of oral contraceptive use. They occur as single, small (≤3 cm in diameter), unilateral subcutaneous nodules near the vulvar vestibule, particularly between the hymen and the pigmented epithelium of the labium minus.

Dilatation of remnants of the vestigial mesonephric ducts, encountered in the lateral aspects of the vulva and, especially, the vagina, results in the rare mesonephric cyst (MNC). MNC at the introitus have been designated as "mesonephric-like" cysts since the mesonephric ducts do not descend to the anlage of the vulva during embryogenesis.

Passing through the inguinal canal, along with the round ligament, to the labium majus is a rudimentary peritoneal sac known as the *canal of Nuck* (processus vaginalis peritonei); persistence and dilatation of the latter results in the infrequent mesothelial cyst (MTC), a structure analogous to the hydrocele of the spermatic cord in males. MTCs are derived from herniation of the peritoneal sac through the inguinal canal at the point where the round ligament inserts into the labium majus.

GROSS

There are no reliable gross appearances to distinguish the aforementioned cysts; however, each has some commonly observed features. Most BCs are filled with a clear, usually sterile, fluid. MCVVs often contain thick, mucoid material. MNCs may have a blue violet hue that causes confusion with cystic endometriosis; however, the fluid within it is clear rather than dark brown and thick. MTCs may be mistaken on gross examination for varicoceles of the vulva as well as inguinal hernias.

HISTOPATHOLOGY

The lining of a BC may be variable and depends on which portion of the glandular or ductular apparatus participates in its formation; thus, one or more cell types may line the cyst and be surrounded by dense, fibroconnective tissue often containing remnants of racemose mucinous glands. The lining may be composed of the following cell types: a typical transitional-type epithelium similar to that present in the normal duct (Fig 11.1); a columnar to cuboidal mucinous epithelium sometimes accompanied by ciliated cells; a compressed and atrophic nonspecific type of epithelium often secondary to longstanding compression atrophy from fluid distention (Fig. 11.2); a partial (Fig. 11.2) or complete squamous lining of metaplastic origin; or a lining completely denuded of epithelium.

MCVVs are found beneath a normal-appearing squamous mucosa and lined by a mucinous type of epithelium similar to that of the mullerian-derived endocervical epithelium (Fig. 11.3); cilia may or may not be present. A single cell lining of cuboidal to tall columnar mucus-producing cells (Fig. 11.4) with pale cytoplasm (mucicarmine, PAS, and Alcian blue–positive) may be thrown into papillary folds or flattened, probably secondary to pressure atrophy from distention with mucus (Fig. 11.3). Squamous metaplasia is common. No well-developed smooth muscle layer is present beneath the epithelium. Similar cysts have been described in the vulvovaginal area of patients treated with 5FU.

MNCs are lined by cuboidal or columnar epithelium without cilia; stains for intracellular mucin and glycogen are negative (Fig. 11.5). The universal presence of a well-developed subepithelial layer of smooth muscle in all MNCs has been questioned; one was not present in the case pictured in Figure 11.5.

MTCs are lined by a single layer of mesothelial cells identical to those lining the rest of the peritoneum; they may exhibit an alarming degree of reactive atypicality (Fig. 11.6).

PROGNOSIS AND TREATMENT

Excisional biopsy of all the cysts described above is often curative; however, some may be associated with easily treatable recurrence.

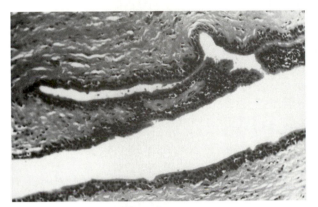

Figure 11.1. Bartholin cyst.

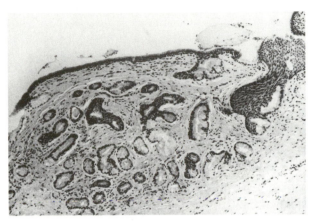

Figure 11.2. Bartholin cyst lined by metaplastic squamous epithelium.

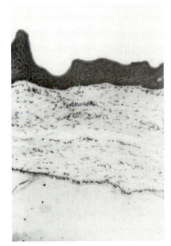

Figure 11.3. Mucus cyst of the vulvar vestibule.

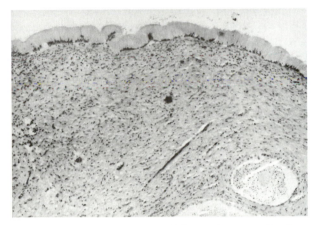

Figure 11.4. Mucus cyst of the vulvar vestibule.

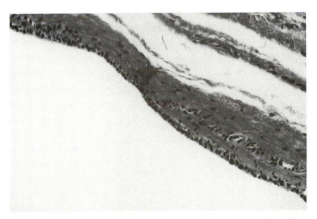

Figure 11.5. Mesonephric cyst-lateral vulvo-vaginal area.

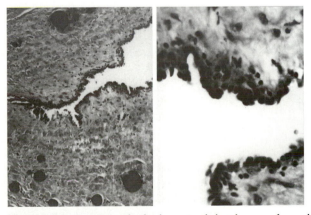

Figure 11.6. Mesothelial cyst of the lower female genital tract.

12. Vulvar Psoriasis
vs.
Lichen Planus
vs.
Seborrheic Dermatitis

CLINICAL

The skin conditions to be discussed in this chapter are so-called papulosquamous diseases, characterized by scaling papules that may coalesce into plaques. Psoriasis (PS) often affects adolescent females, beginning around age 16. Indeed, almost 20% of patients have their first episode around the menarche, a quarter of them at their first pregnancy, and another quarter at the menopause. PS rarely may be localized to the outer labia majora and genitocrural areas, but more often the lesions affect the intertriginous areas of the groin, intergluteal folds, and axillae.

Lichen planus (LP) is rarely confined to the vulva in middle-aged females. It affects both the skin and the mucous membranes of the vulva; indeed, the presence of vulvar mucosal lesions should prompt a search for oral ones.

Seborrheic dermatitis (SD) affects skin with a high concentration of sebaceous glands and may involve the genital and perianal skin, particularly in obese women, usually sparing the labia minora.

GROSS

Uncomplicated lesions of genital PS appear as symmetrical, dull red papular eruptions, with sharply defined borders and a covering of fine silvery scales, which may coalesce to form plaques. Because of the moist environment, scaling may be minimal or absent.

The lesions of LP typically appear as discrete or confluent well-defined, slightly raised, flat-topped polygonal papules or as a delicate, interlacing network of bluish to white reticulate lines, a manifestation that is particularly common when the mucous membranes of the vestibule or inner aspects of the labia minora are affected.

Vulvar SD typically appears as erythematous, sharply defined plaques covered by fine, yellow to red, often greasy, nonadherent scales in contrast to the silvery scales of PS.

HISTOPATHOLOGY

The appearance of PS varies with the age of the lesion, and all the classic features are not often encountered in a single biopsy. However, in well-established lesions of PS the following are often seen: prominent epidermal psoriasiform hyperplasia with elongation and clubbing of the rete pegs (Fig. 12.1), a mitotically active basal and parabasal cell layer, acanthosis, parakeratosis with an absent or markedly diminished granular cell layer (Fig. 12.2), thinning of the suprapapillary plates, elongation of the dermal papillae with edema, dilated and tortuous dermal capillaries with extravasated red blood cells, accumulation of neutrophilic aggregates (Munro's microabscesses) in the parakeratotic horny layer of the stratum corneum (Fig. 12.3), and dermal perivascular inflammation.

In uncomplicated cases of LP, the characteristic microscopic changes include the following features: acanthosis and irregular elongation of the rete ridges (Fig. 12.4), many of which exhibit pointed basal aspects imparting an overall "sawtoothed" appearance of the squamous epithelium; hyperkeratosis and an increased granular cell layer (Fig. 12.4); a dense band-like infiltrate of lymphocytes that apposes and tightly hugs the dermal–epithelial junction (Fig. 12.4); inflammatory infiltration of the overlying squamous epithelium accompanied by liquefactive degeneration or destruction of the basal layer, resulting in obscurement and haziness of the dermal–epithelial junction (Fig. 12.5); and the presence of degenerated cells or colloid bodies within the squamous epithelium. Particularly in mucosal lesions of vulvar LP, the histology may be quite nonspecific, but the presence of liquefactive degeneration and destruction of the basal layer may be especially helpful in suggesting the proper diagnosis.

The epidermis of SD exhibits a mild to moderate acanthosis, some elongation, and clubbing of rete ridges, without thinning of the suprapapillary plates and the dilated capillary vessels typical of PS. In early lesions a spongiotic dermatitis typically shows foci of parakeratosis containing neutrophils (Fig. 12.6), especially in the region of the follicular infundibulum (but no Monro's microabscesses). The superficial dermis often contains a sparse perivascular mononuclear inflammatory infiltrate. Chronic lesions no longer display spongiosis, and the epidermis assumes a psoriasiform pattern of hyperplasia.

PROGNOSIS AND TREATMENT

Various forms of corticosteroids have been a mainstay of treatment for vulvar PS, LP, and SD; additionally, topical or ingested psoralens followed by ultraviolet light (PUVA) have also been used successfully to treat PS; however, the latter are difficult to use with genital lesions.

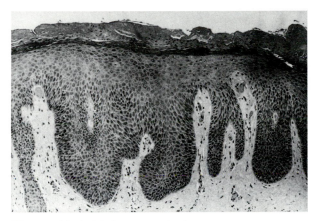

Figure 12.1. Vulvar psoriasis.

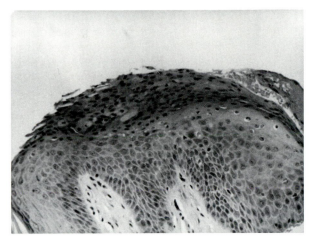

Figure 12.2. Vulvar psoriasis.

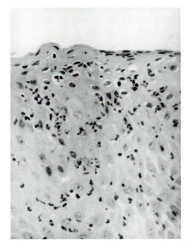

Figure 12.3. Vulvar psoriasis.

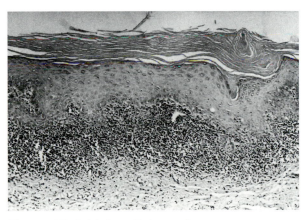

Figure 12.4. Vulvar lichen planus.

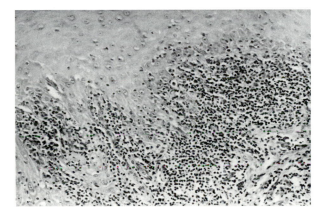

Figure 12.5. Vulvar lichen planus.

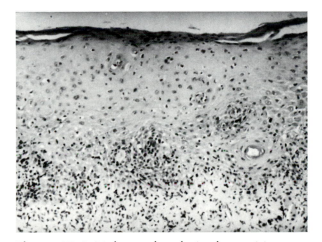

Figure 12.6. Vulvar seborrheic dermatitis.

13. Superficially Invasive Squamous Carcinoma vs. High-Grade VIN with Pseudoinvasion

CLINICAL

There are few specific clinical findings that aid in the distinction of the patient with superficially invasive squamous carcinoma (SIVC) from one with only high-grade vulvar intraepithelial neoplasia (VIN). Because of the relatively capricious biologic behavior of superficially invasive vulvar squamous cancers, the term "microinvasive" squamous carcinoma is no longer recommended. Such carcinomas are included within stage IA tumors, as recently defined by the International Federation of Gynecology and Obstetrics (FIGO) and the International Society for the study of Vulvar Disease: lesions 2 cm or less in size confined to the vulva or perineum and with stromal invasion no greater than 1.0 mm (no nodal metastasis). The depth of invasion is measured from the epithelial-stromal junction of the adjacent most superficial dermal papillae to the deepest point of invasion.

GROSS

SIVC may present as an ulcer, as a white hyperkeratotic plaque, as an erythematous papule or macule, or as an area of hyperpigmentation with a brown or black hue; there are no reliable gross features that distinguish SIVC from high-grade VIN.

HISTOPATHOLOGY

Probably the earliest and most consistently recognizable cytologic feature of a SIVC arising from a VIN is an increase in the amount of eosinophilic cytoplasm in the cells of the former; indeed, when this phenomenon is observed in a VIN without initial evidence of invasion, deeper sections are in order to rule out concomitant SIVC. The earliest architectural evidence of invasion is a small tongue-like bud of cells, with increased eosinophilic cytoplasm, protruding into the stroma but still connected to the overlying VIN (Fig. 13.1). Some other histopathologic features of unequivocal SIVC include the following: change in the nature of chromatin from coarse hyperchromatism and less prominent nucleoli of high-grade VIN to open, vesicular, cleared chromatin (Fig. 13.1) and prominent nucleoli of SIVC; isolated single cells or small, irregularly shaped nests of cells in the subepithelial stroma (Figs. 13.2, 13.3); lack of the orderly peripheral palisading of cells (characteristically present in the basal aspects of VIN) at the border of tumor nests with the stroma (Figs. 13.2, 13.3); and the presence of a stromal response in the form of edematous loos-

ening and desmoplasia around tumor nests (Figs. 13.2, 13.3). In more equivocal cases of stromal invasion, the possibility of pseudoinvasion secondary to tangential sectioning of high-grade VIN must be considered. Particular care must be exercised in the interpretation of specimens removed from the hairbearing portions of the vulva since up to two-thirds of cases of VIN involve the pilosebaceous structures. Such pilosebaceous units replaced with high-grade VIN often appear to be free-lying in the dermis and totally separate from the overlying epidermis; the resultant appearance may be highly suggestive of SIVC (Fig. 13.4). Deeper cuts into the block will often reveal the nature of the lesion and its connection with the epidermis. Additionally, both polypoid and flat types of VIN lesions are notoriously complex in their architecture, with bulky rete pegs exhibiting markedly irregular sizes and shapes; on tangential sectioning, similar complex folds in the basal aspects of both can engender apparent nests of free-lying tumor in the dermis. This situation may present more of a problem in differentiated types of VIN, raising the question of well-differentiated SIVC. Careful examination will usually reveal no stromal response to such nests of pseudoinvasive tumor, and the edges of the nests will often display either a sharp, "crisp" border with the surrounding stroma (Fig. 13.5), often accompanied by peripheral palisading of cells at the epithelial–stromal border, or sometimes a "fuzziness" that should raise the question of tangential sectioning. It should be noted, however, that superficially invasive nests may actually arise from the bases of such architecturally complex extensions of VIN III into the stroma (Fig. 13.6). Since 90% of high-grade VIN lesions are said to exhibit infiltrates of lymphocytes, plasma cells, and histiocytes, their presence probably is of limited usefulness in the distinction of true invasion from pseudoinvasion.

High-grade VIN may also extend into the major and minor vestibular glands of the vulva as well as into the periurethral glands. Tangential sectioning of VIN-replaced glandular clefts may likewise simulate nests of invasive squamous carcinoma.

PROGNOSIS AND TREATMENT

The prognosis of vulvar SIVC is relatively good. Most workers regard wide local excision to be adequate treatment if (1) a thorough and accurate pathologic examination has been accomplished, revealing, in particular, an absence of vascular space invasion and (2) groin nodes are not suspiciously enlarged. In the face of suspicious groin nodes, an ipsilateral node dissection often is considered to be adequate.

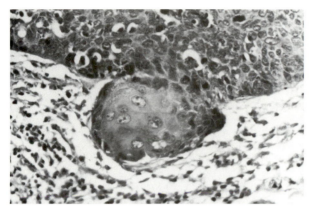

Figure 13.1. Superficially invasive vulvar squamous carcinoma, earliest phase.

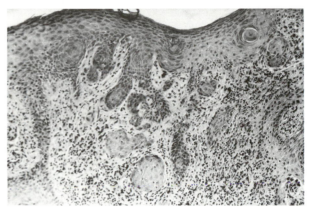

Figure 13.2. Superficially invasive vulvar squamous carcinoma.

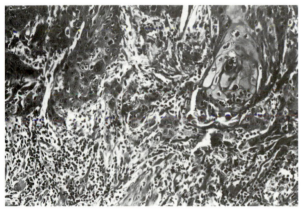

Figure 13.3. Superficially invasive vulvar squamous carcinoma.

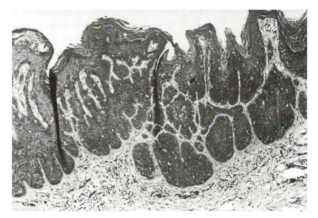

Figure 13.4. VIN III with tangentially sectioned irregular dermal-epidermal junction ("pseudoinvasion").

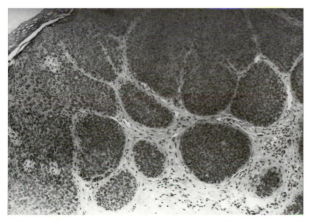

Figure 13.5. VIN III with tangentially sectioned irregular dermal-epidermal junction ("pseudoinvasion").

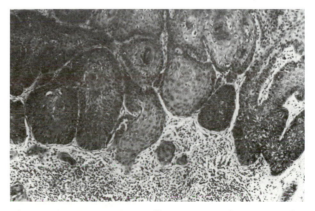

Figure 13.6. Tangentially sectioned VIN III also with foci of superficial invasion of squamous cell carcinoma.

Section 2

VAGINAL DISORDERS

14. Rhabdomyoma

vs.

Embryonal Rhabdomyosarcoma ("Sarcoma Botryoides")

CLINICAL

Despite their rarity in the routine practice of surgical pathology, the clinical and pathologic distinction between rhabdomyoma (RH) and embryonal rhabdomyosarcoma (ER) is of paramount importance to prevent misdiagnosis and improper treatment.

The vagina is the most common site of genital RH. Most of these rhabdomyomas arise from the anterior or posterior vaginal wall in middle-aged women and are usually asymptomatic. ER is the most common vaginal sarcoma and the most frequently encountered neoplasm in the lower urogenital tract of infants and young girls; indeed, two-thirds of ER arise within the first 2 years of life. Most arise from the anterior vaginal wall affecting the vesicovaginal septum and the posterior bladder wall.

GROSS

Vaginal RHs may range from 1 to 10 cm in diameter but are often single, small, pale tan, and multilobated with a glistening surface. In contrast, ERs often present as multiple, polypoid, pedunculated tumors that fill the vaginal vault and protrude from the introitus. They may appear edematous or myxomatous and display a glistening, translucent white to gray surface appearance.

HISTOPATHOLOGY

In a vaginal RH, the squamous mucosa is usually intact and relatively normal (Fig. 14.1), as is often the case with ER. The underlying stroma in a RH is often loose and delicate and sometimes myxoid (particularly common in the "fetal myxoid" type that tends to occur in the genital tract). Often deep within the polypoid RH are more elongated, eosinophilic strap cells, derived from striated muscle, in which cross-striations are quite evident. Immature mesenchymal cells are a rarity in RH but diffusely present in ER. Mature strap cells tend to be arranged in broad, interlacing bundles (Fig. 14.2—left) and are usually thinner in width than normal striated muscle. Interspersed among them are uniformly larger rhabdomyoblastic-type cells with copious eosinophilic cytoplasm and large, centrally or eccentrically located nuclei (Fig. 14.2—right). Nucleoli may be prominent, but significant nu-

clear atypicality or mitotic activity are not features; the latter two features are often prominent in ER.

The polypoid excrescences of ER (Fig. 14.3) are composed of primitive-appearing, mitotically active, poorly differentiated mesenchymal cells originating from the lamina propria; such cells may be sparse and set in a loose myxoid stroma. Interspersed among more elongate strap cells of ER, small, round cells with dense nuclei and little cytoplasm (Fig. 14.4) may easily be confused with inflammatory cells. Their tendency to condense around blood vessels may help differentiate them from benign round cell infiltrates but not from lymphoid tumors.

ERs may exhibit three relatively distinctive-appearing histologic zones. The most characteristic microscopic feature of ER is represented by a zone of densely cellular sarcoma immediately beneath the normal but thinned squamous epithelium, the "cambium layer" (shown in Fig. 14.5), which some feel is virtually pathognomonic of the entity. Deep within this zone is a paucicellular myxoid stroma of banal appearing spindled to stellate-shaped cells (Fig. 14.5). A biopsy comprised largely of this zone may cause confusion with a benign entity. In the deepest aspect of the tumor one may easily find "strap" cells, some of which exhibit the characteristic cross-striations of ER (Fig. 14.6). Some claim that islands of mature cartilage may be seen. Because of the tendency toward histologic zonation, the diagnosis of ER on biopsy may be difficult, and interpretation may depend on the portion of the tumor from which the biopsy was taken.

Immunostains may aid in the diagnosis of ER. Myoglobin is specific for striated muscle and may be useful in the identification of immature rhabdomyoblasts that are either sparsely present or are so immature or poorly differentiated that cross-striations are not evident by light microscopy. Approximately 60–90% of ERs will be positive for myoglobin, depending on the degree of differentiation of the primitive skeletal muscle element.

PROGNOSIS AND TREATMENT

Vaginal RHs are benign tumors treated by local excision. The current prognosis in ER is much better, due to less radical surgery (sparing rectum and bladder) and the use of multimodality therapy. Pelvic recurrences are common, and the cause of death is more commonly related to direct extension than from distant metastases.

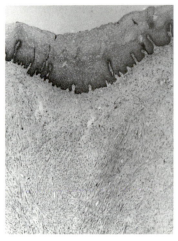

Figure 14.1. Vaginal rhabdomyoma.

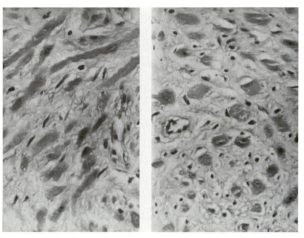

Figure 14.2. Vaginal rhabdomyoma.

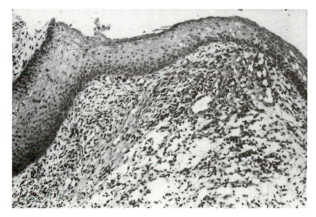

Figure 14.3. Embryonal rhabdomyosarcoma ("sarcoma botryoides") arising from the vaginal wall.

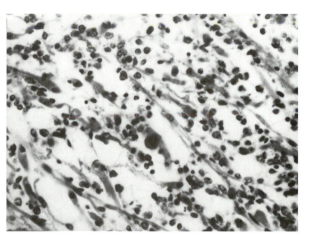

Figure 14.4. Vaginal embryonal rhabdomyosarcoma ("sarcoma botryoides").

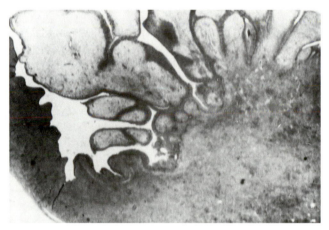

Figure 14.5. Vaginal embryonal rhabdomyosarcoma ("sarcoma botryoides").

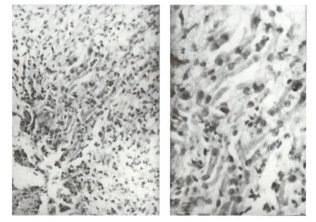

Figure 14.6. Vaginal embryonal rhabdomyosarcoma ("sarcoma botryoides").

15. Embryonal Rhabdomyosarcoma ("Sarcoma Botryoides")

vs.

Vaginal Pseudosarcomatous Polyp ("Pseudosarcoma Botryoides")

vs.

Aggressive Angiomyxoma

CLINICAL

The clinical characteristics of embryonal rhabdomyosarcoma (ER) are covered in Chapter 14. Pseudosarcomatous vaginal polyps (PSVPs) are rare. Occurring largely in women older than 20, they may be hormone-related (about a third occur in pregnancy). Most are single and arise from the lower-third left lateral vaginal wall. Most PSVPs are incidental findings and do not have the clinical history of rapid growth typical of ER.

Aggressive angiomyxoma (AA) is rare and usually encountered in the soft tissues of the vulva, vagina, and perineal area of young women in their 2nd and 3rd decades. It is slow-growing and may be confused clinically with a Bartholin cyst when it arises in the vulvovaginal area.

GROSS

The gross characteristics of ER are discussed in Chapter 14. Most PSVPs are polypoid or pedunculated, and some are finger-like masses. The median diameter is 2 cm, and PSVPs appear gray to white on section, with a soft or rubbery consistency.

Aggressive angiomyxoma is usually a large, and sometimes polypoid lesion, most often >10 cm in diameter. AA may extend from the vulvovaginal soft tissues into the ischiorectal fossa and the retroperitoneum. On cut section, AA has a uniform, glistening, gelatinous to myxoid appearance; it usually has a relatively poorly defined margin with its surrounding soft tissues.

HISTOPATHOLOGY

The histopathologic aspects of ER are discussed in Chapter 14. Like ER, PVSPs are covered by a normal but attenuated vaginal squamous epithelium (Figs. 15.1, 15.2). The connective-tissue core is loose and focally edematous with abundant capillary-sized vessels. Extensive edema is not a striking feature. Importantly, although the stromal core may be cellular, there is no hypercellular subepithelial "cambium layer" typical of ER (Fig. 15.1). Mitoses are infrequent (rarely more than 3 mitotic figures per 10 high-power fields). Although abnormal mitotic figures are only rarely encountered in PVSPs, they do occur (Fig. 15.2) and can further contribute to confusion with ER when present. Approximately half of PSVPs contain large, bizarre epithelioid to spindle-shaped stromal cells that probably are derived from atypical fibroblasts (Figs. 15.2, 15.3); some workers have noted their resemblance to "radiation-type fibroblasts." Nuclei are often single, but multinucleation is not uncommon. Despite the associated nuclear hyperchromatism and pleomorphism, histologic features of malignancy such as coarse chromatin clumping and high nucleoplasmic ratio are not evident. Delicate, pointed cytoplasmic processes are often seen (Fig. 15.3), but intracytoplasmic cross-striations are not a feature. Neither small undifferentiated stromal cells nor rhabdomyoblasts are seen, and there is no invasion of the intact overlying squamous epithelium, as is typical of ER.

AAs are composed of abundant, loose myxoid stroma alternating with a prominent, densely collagenous element (Fig. 15.4). Within the stroma are scattered stellate to spindle-shaped tumor cells with small, monotonous, densely hyperchromatic nuclei and small nucleoli. Nuclei are bland and pleomorphism is not significant (Figs. 15.5, 15.6). AAs are highly vascular and contain abundant variably-sized blood vessels. Capillaries and variable caliber (often medium-sized) arteries and veins with medial hypertrophy are particularly prominent (Figs. 15.5—arrow, 15.6) and are frequently widely ectatic with extravasated red cells. Brisk mitotic activity as well as other features of malignancy such as necrosis are lacking; however, careful examination and proper sampling at the advancing edge of the tumor often will reveal histologic evidence of skeletal muscle or adipose tissue invasion. Occasionally, glandular elements may be present, and the latter must be differentiated from those entrapped by the invading neoplasm.

PROGNOSIS AND TREATMENT

The prognosis and treatment of ERs are discussed in Chapter 14. PSVP is a benign lesion adequately treated with excision or reexicision in the event of incomplete removal. The current treatment for AA is as complete a surgical excision as is technically possible. Although there is a high frequency of local recurrence, the latter may be due to inadequate excision since all patients appear to be alive and well following surgical reexcision.

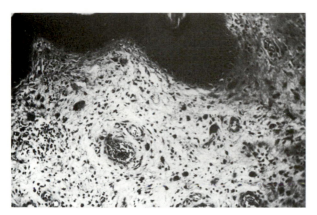

Figure 15.1. Vaginal pseudosarcomatous polyp.

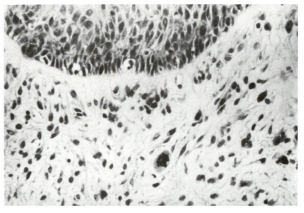

Figure 15.2. Vaginal pseudosarcomatous polyp containing an abnormal mitotic figure in the stroma.

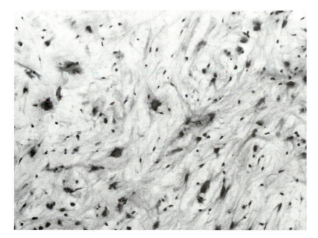

Figure 15.3. Vaginal pseudosarcomatous polyp.

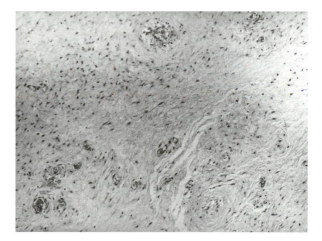

Figure 15.4. Aggressive angiomyxoma-vagina.

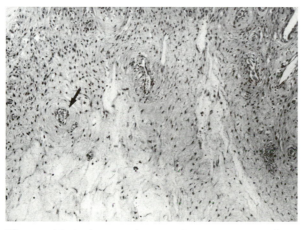

Figure 15.5. Aggressive angiomyxoma-vagina.

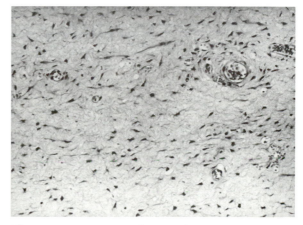

Figure 15.6. Aggressive angiomyxoma-vagina.

16. Mullerian Papilloma

vs.

Prolapsed Fallopian Tube Postvaginal Hysterectomy

vs.

Recurrent Papillary Endometrial or Ovarian Carcinoma

CLINICAL

The mullerian papilloma (MP) typically occurs in infants and young girls, between the ages of 2 and 5, with vaginal bleeding or discharge. On pelvic examination the mucosa of the cervix or upper vagina exhibits an exophytic papillary lesion.

Eighty percent of prolapsed fallopian tubes (PFT) follow a vaginal hysterectomy, most often within 6 months. Patients may complain of abdominal pain; vaginal bleeding; watery, foul discharge; or severe dyspareunia.

Although primary carcinoma of the vagina is extremely rare, recurrence of either endometrial or ovarian carcinoma at the vaginal apex is encountered relatively commonly, particularly in older women. Many recurrent tumors are detected because of symptomatic vaginal bleeding or discharge or at a routine clinical posttreatment follow-up examination.

GROSS

The MP, the PFT, and recurrent carcinoma may appear quite similar, all having the ability to present as an exophytic, polypoid, or papillary lesion with a red, granular appearance. On close examination, particularly with the aid of a colposcope, the fact that the "papillae" of a PFT are actually tubal fimbriae may actually be discerned.

HISTOPATHOLOGY

Mullerian papilloma consists of multiple, rather delicate papillary fronds (Fig. 16.1); the papillae are of various sizes and shapes and consist of fibrovascular cores of variably dense connective tissue lined by a benign-appearing glandular epithelium (Fig. 16.2). The stromal cores may be loose and myxomatous, raising the ques-

tion of ER. The fibrovascular papillary cores are lined by cuboidal to low or tall columnar glandular epithelium (Fig. 16.3), although in some cases the cells are more flattened. In others a hobnail appearance reminiscent of clear cell carcinoma may be imparted but clear cells and intracellular glycogen may be absent. At the bases of the papillae, congeries of complex cribriform glands with a microglandular type of architectural pattern may be present and further mimic clear cell carcinoma. Finally, however, there is neither sufficient cytologic atypicality nor mitotic activity to support a malignant diagnosis. A mucinous type of differentiation, reminiscent of endocervical epithelium, is evident in some, but certainly not all, MPs; the latter supports the currently held theory that MPs are of mullerian, rather than mesonephric origin, as was once believed. Most cases exhibit some degree of squamous metaplasia.

In a PFT, the architecture of the tubal plicae and fimbriae may have been mechanically distorted and obscured by considerable edema, a dense acute and chronic inflammatory infiltrate and granulation tissue (Fig. 16.4). The glandular epithelium may show a worrisome and reactive inflammatory atypia, sometimes accompanied by an architecturally complex and worrisome pseudomalignant phenomenon (Fig. 16.5) that is well known to occur in severely inflamed tubes. The chance for a diagnostic error is enhanced by the prior suggestion of severe atypia or malignancy on cervicovaginal smear since such cells can shed into the vaginal pool and be sampled. The histologic findings, when not too obscured, of typical-appearing tubal cytology and architecture, including the presence of organized bundles of smooth muscle around hyperplastic tubal-type epithelium, should suffice to avoid misdiagnosis. The observation of ciliated columnar cells in an atypical cervicovaginal smear, particularly in the face of a clinically evident papillary vaginal lesion, should raise the question of tubal epithelium and prompt a call to the clinician about the possibility of a PFT.

Both recurrent endometrial and ovarian adenocarcinoma often occur in papillary forms (Fig. 16.6—left) but are associated with obviously malignant cytologic and architectural features peculiar to their parent tumor type. The latter includes brisk mitotic activity, nuclear pleomorphism, and nuclear hyperchromatism (Fig. 16.6—right).

PROGNOSIS AND TREATMENT

MPs are benign and eliminated by complete surgical excision. PFTs are treated by complete excision through the vaginal cuff since electrocautery is ineffective treatment. Recurrent endometrial or ovarian adenocarcinomas are treated by ancillary therapy.

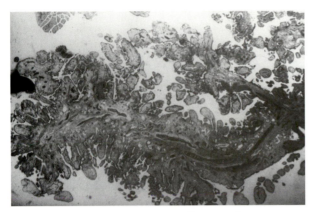

Figure 16.1. Mullerian papilloma of vagina.

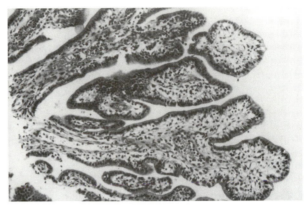

Figure 16.2. Mullerian papilloma of vagina.

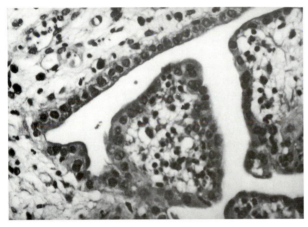

Figure 16.3. Mullerian papilloma of vagina.

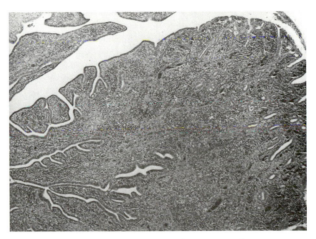

Figure 16.4. "Prolapsed" fallopian tube post vaginal hysterectomy.

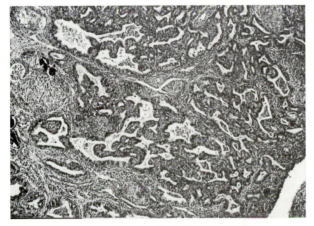

Figure 16.5. "Prolapsed" fallopian tube post vaginal hysterectomy with pseudocarcinomatous changes.

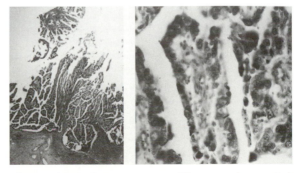

Figure 16.6. Recurrent papillary endometrial adenocarcinoma in vaginal vault.

17. Postoperative Spindle Cell Nodule (Vaginal Vault) vs.

Primary Vaginal Sarcoma [Excluding Embryonal Rhabdomyosarcoma ("Sarcoma Botryoides")]

CLINICAL

Postoperative spindle cell nodule (PSCN) is a relatively recently recognized entity that involves the genitourinary tract, including the urinary bladder, urethra, and vagina. Occurring from 5 weeks to 3 months postoperatively, PSCN should be strongly considered when a mass develops following either a biopsy, surgery, or trauma. Indeed, the absence of such a clinical history would militate against the diagnosis of PSCN.

Excluding ER, primary vaginal sarcomas (PVS) account for less than 2% of all malignant vaginal tumors. PVSs often present with abnormal vaginal bleeding in women in their 4th decade. In one study approximately a third of patients who developed a PVS had a prior history of radiation therapy for cervical carcinoma. Of all reported PVSs, 30–60% are leiomyosarcomas, an important observation since the PSCN is most commonly confused with a malignant smooth muscle tumor.

GROSS

Generally, PSCNs are considerably smaller than primary VSs. Virtually all of PSCNs are submucosal in location, are <4 cm in maximum diameter, and obviously tend to occur at the previous surgery site.

Primary VSs, in contrast to PSCNs, are frequently large, bulky tumors that elicit a clinical suspicion of cancer. Some VSs are relatively small and may overlap in size with PSCN; however, the typical VS is ≥10 cm in maximum diameter. Most exhibit a cut surface with a firm, fish-flesh consistency typical of many other types of sarcomas. Few are encapsulated, and an infiltrative growth pattern may be appreciated.

HISTOPATHOLOGY

PSCNs frequently develop immediately beneath the vaginal squamous epithelium and are commonly accompanied by ulceration (Fig. 17.1) because of the tenuous nature of the overlying squamous mucosa. They are often highly cellular and composed of interlacing bundles or fascicles of spindle-shaped cells with plump, eosinophilic to amphophilic cytoplasm (Figs. 17.2, 17.3). PSCNs may display an alarming degree of mitotic activity (reportedly up to 25 per 10 high-power fields). In more mature lesions the rate may be much lower, on the order of 1–2 per 10 high-power fields (Fig. 17.3). A disturbing histologic feature is the ability of the lesion to project an infiltrative appearance in the surrounding soft tissues. Because of their aforementioned increased cellularity, brisk mitotic activity, and prominent nucleoli, a diagnosis of VS is often seriously entertained; the most frequent considerations are leiomyosarcoma and malignant fibrous histiocytoma, because of the tendency of the PSCN to form interlacing bundles and fascicles of whorled cells or a cartwheel-type pattern (Fig. 17.4). The extensive, delicate capillary network in the background of the lesion, commonly accompanied by stromal hemorrhage, can impart a histologic appearance disturbingly similar to Kaposi's sarcoma (Fig. 17.5); the latter is manifested by extravasated red blood cells in slit-like spaces. Most of the proliferating cells are either reactive fibroblasts, myofibroblasts, smooth muscle cells, or combinations of those cell types. Despite the aforementioned worrisome findings, the nuclear features are not those of a sarcoma; in fact, the nuclei are quite uniform in size and shape with delicate, finely dispersed chromatin and one or two distinct nucleoli. Hyperchromatism and pleomorphism are not features, and any evidence of such should cast doubt on the diagnosis of PSCN.

Leiomyosarcoma (LMS), the most commonly encountered VS, has the same histopathologic appearance as in other body sites, typified by a highly cellular neoplasm with significant nuclear atypicality and brisk mitotic activity (Fig. 17.6). Many workers feel that the degree of mitotic activity is the single most useful predictor of prognosis. Some have proposed that smooth muscle tumors with greater than 5 mitotic figures per 10 high-power fields, and either moderate or marked cellular atypicality be classified as leiomyosarcomas. Mitotic activity and nuclear atypicality appear to be more common in recurrent smooth muscle tumors.

PROGNOSIS AND TREATMENT

PSCNs are adequately treated by simple local excision. Despite their disturbing appearance, particularly when they occur in patients who have a previous history of genital tract cancer, they have a completely benign clinical course. Recurrences are likely secondary to incomplete excision. Overt vaginal leiomyosarcomas tend to invade and recur locally. They are treated surgically, but the 5-year survival in one study was only 36%.

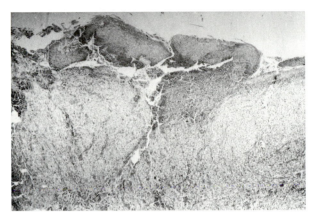

Figure 17.1. Postoperative spindle cell nodule-vaginal vault.

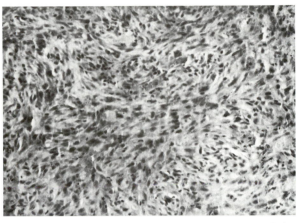

Figure 17.2. Postoperative spindle cell nodule-vaginal vault.

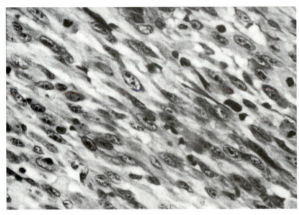

Figure 17.3. Postoperative spindle cell nodule-vaginal vault.

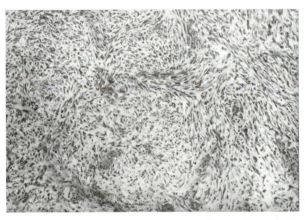

Figure 17.4. Postoperative spindle cell nodule-vaginal vault.

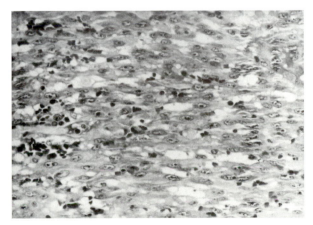

Figure 17.5. Postoperative spindle cell nodule-vaginal vault.

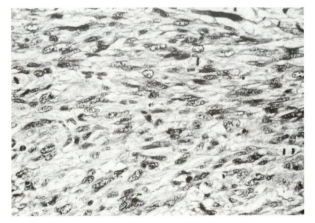

Figure 17.6. Primary vaginal sarcoma (leiomyosarcoma).

18. Secondary Malignant Mixed Mesodermal Tumor (Endometrial or Ovarian) vs. Benign Mixed Tumor vs. Sarcomatoid (Spindle Cell) Squamous Carcinoma

CLINICAL

Secondary vaginal neoplasia represents over 90% of all vaginal adenocarcinomas and endometrial cancers represent roughly one-third of them; one study showed 20% of uterine malignant mixed mesodermal tumors (MMMTs) to have metastasized or spread contiguously to the vagina at the time of death.

The benign mixed tumor of the vagina (BMT) is rare and occurs in relatively younger women (mean age 31 years) than MMMTs (mean age 65 years). BMTs are often asymptomatic and incidental findings on pelvic exam.

Most sarcomatoid carcinomas (SCCs) that involve the vagina are secondary, often from the cervix.

GROSS

Metastases of MMMT from the uterus usually occur on the upper third anterior vaginal wall. So-called surface implants are more commonly encountered as discrete nodules having a predilection for the anterior and lower third of the vagina.

The BMT frequently appears as a 1.5–5-cm polypoid, pale gray to pink submucosal mass or masses near the hymenal ring; BMTs are discrete and well circumscribed but nonencapsulated and are usually covered by a normal appearing squamous mucosa. On cut section, the surface is pale gray to pink without evidence of hemorrhage or necrosis.

The sarcomatoid variant of vaginal SCC appears to have no reliably consistent gross features peculiar to the entity.

HISTOPATHOLOGY

Metastatic MMMT is known for its histopathologic variability; a third of MMMTs are mixtures of clearly malig-

nant epithelial and mesenchymal elements typified by the carcinosarcoma illustrated in Figure 18.1.

Low-power examination of a BMT of the vagina reveals a relatively normal overlying squamous mucosa and a sharp, well-demarcated border with the adjacent vaginal stroma (Fig. 18.2). BMTs frequently consist of mixtures of epithelial and mesenchymal tissues. Moderately to markedly cellular combinations of stroma, variable amounts of admixed squamous epithelium (Figs. 18.3—arrow, 18.4) and, less commonly, glandular epithelium are typically encountered. The stromal element often predominates (Fig. 18.3) and is made up of small, spindle-shaped cells typically arranged in whorled bundles and intersecting fascicles. Nuclei are oval and bland with finely granular chromatin and often small, indistinct nucleoli. Mitotic figures are characteristically uncommon, but in one study about one-fourth of cases exhibited significant mitotic activity. The spindled stroma surrounds well-delineated nests and islands of mature squamous epithelium (Fig. 18.4) that may show prominent glycogenation, keratinization, and even pearl formation. Merging with the squamous epithelium is randomly interspersed mucinous-type epithelium that occasionally forms small glands (Fig. 18.4) lined by simple cuboidal to flattened epithelium. The combination of mucinous and squamous epithelium sometimes may impart an appearance that resembles endocervical glandular mucosa associated with squamous metaplasia (Fig. 18.4), or a Brenner tumor of the ovary. Another frequent observation is the presence of droplets or cytoplasmic pools of mucin, often within the squamous epithelium. The various combinations of cellular stroma combined with squamous and glandular epithelia may lead to the erroneous diagnosis of a malignant mixed mesodermal tumor. Although atypia is not a characteristic feature of BMTs of the vagina, occasionally there is worrisome nuclear atypia, which, in combination with the aforementioned occasional brisk mitotic activity and infiltrative-appearing borders, may, indeed, raise the legitimate question of malignancy.

On low-power examination, the pseudosarcomatous component of a sarcomatoid SCC often merges imperceptibly with the more easily recognizable squamous component (Fig. 18.5). In other sarcomatoid SCCs, the squamous element is present in the form of small, compact pearls within the spindled and pseudosarcomatous component (Fig. 18.6). In one study of SCC, although the highly pleomorphic pseudosarcomatous spindled cell pattern was predominant, each tumor had a component of moderately well-differentiated SCC associated with it. The latter points out the fact that a small biopsy may miss the more readily identifiable squamous component; immunostains for cytokeratins, in particular, may elucidate the nature of any sarcomatoid areas.

PROGNOSIS AND TREATMENT

The prognosis for high stage MMMT is poor, and there is still no effective chemotherapy for advanced disease and recurrent MMMT. The typical forms of BMT of the vagina have been cured by simple local surgical excision, and those that have exhibited atypia and infiltrative-appearing borders have likewise, to date, shown no signs of recurrence or metastasis. The treatment for sarcomatoid SCC is no different from that for any other poorly differentiated SCC.

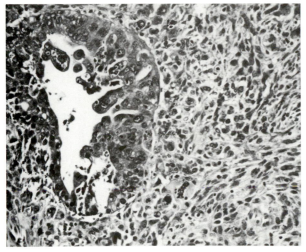

Figure 18.1. Recurrent endometrial malignant mixed mesodermal tumor-vaginal vault.

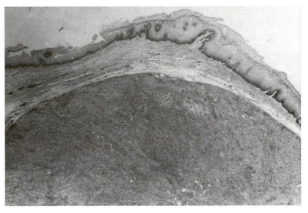

Figure 18.2. Benign mixed tumor of the vagina.

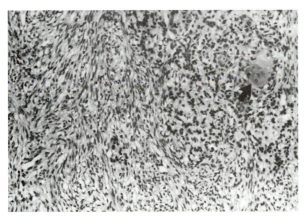

Figure 18.3. Benign mixed tumor of the vagina.

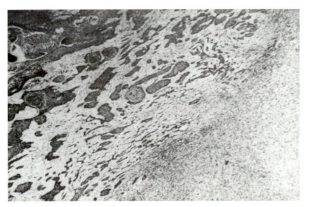

Figure 18.4. Benign mixed tumor of the vagina.

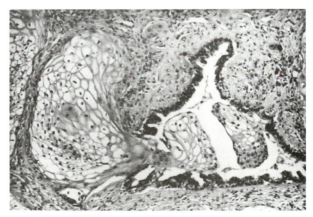

Figure 18.5. Sarcomatoid (spindle cell) squamous carcinoma of the vagina.

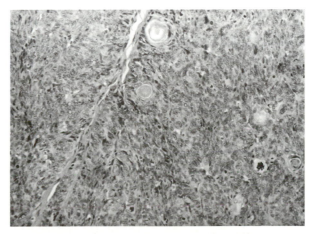

Figure 18.6. Sarcomatoid (spindle cell) squamous carcinoma of the vagina.

19. Radiation-induced Squamous Atypia
vs.
Vaginal Intraepithelial Neoplasia (VAIN)

CLINICAL

Radiation therapy used in the treatment of cervical cancer exposes the vagina to low-level doses leading to radiation-induced persistent atypia as well as postradiation dysplasia. Approximately a third of women with VAIN have had a prior history of ionizing radiation.

Non-radiation-associated VAIN usually occurs as part of the spectrum of squamous intraepithelial lesions known as the "lower female genital tract neoplasia syndrome"; the latter arises from a multicentric "field effect" within the anogenital area, vagina, and cervix secondary to infection with human papilloma virus (HPV).

GROSS

There are no macroscopic findings that permit the distinction of persistent radiation-induced atypia from postradiation VAIN or ordinary VAIN; however, the former would more likely be present in the background of a relatively atrophic-appearing mucosa. In the latter two, the characteristic colposcopic features of mosaicism and punctation are similar to those of the cervix.

HISTOPATHOLOGY

Following irradiation, ulceration, and reepithelialization, the vaginal squamous epithelium appears better developed after 2 years, but never has the appearance of a normal stratified squamous epithelium. In so-called persistent radiation-induced atypia (PRA), the nuclei of the squamous epithelial cells may show slight and persistent enlargement (Fig. 19.1); further, their cytoplasm, although relatively abundant, may exhibit vacuolization and raise the question, particularly at low magnification, of a low-grade HPV effect (Fig. 19.1). In other cases of PRA the squamous cell nuclei may exhibit more atypicality, manifested by more pleomorphism, greater hyperchromatism (Fig. 19.2), and isolated, bizarre nuclei that are abnormally large compared to their neighbors; however, higher-power examination most often shows the chromatin to be smudged and degenerative-appearing (Figs. 19.2, 19.3) rather than irregularly and coarsely clumped as is seen in true high-grade VAIN. Such

changes may persist for years after therapy. As mentioned above, binucleation (Fig. 19.3) and perinuclear halos, changes similar to those seen with HPV effect, may occur. Small nucleoli may be present. In some examples of PRA, the underlying connective-tissue stromal changes are more dramatic, displaying the characteristic appearance of radiation damage manifested by hyalinization, bizarre "radiation-type" fibroblasts, microscopic areas of necrosis, vascular ectasia (Fig. 19.4), and extravasation of red cells into the stroma (Fig. 19.5—arrows). An infiltrate of chronic inflammatory cells, usually in the form of lymphocytes and plasma cells, is common. However, such changes should be separated from so-called postirradiation dysplasia, which may occur after a latent period ranging from months to years. The intraepithelial changes in postirradiation dysplasia are similar to those of ordinary VAIN and consist of varying degrees of maturational disturbance, corresponding to VAIN I, II, and III; the aforementioned characteristic stromal changes usually remain. Hyperkeratosis may be present, and often there is a well-defined granular cell layer. Perinuclear halos are quite common in persistent irradiation dysplasia, a fact that has led some to postulate reactivation of latent HPV as a factor in their genesis.

The histopathologic diagnosis of ordinary VAIN may be based on a three-grade system (VAIN I, II, III) similar to that used in the diagnosis of vulvar and cervical intraepithelial squamous neoplasia. Alternatively, one may employ a binary system similar to that used in the Bethesda system, recognizing low-grade and high-grade (Fig. 19.6) squamous intraepithelial lesions; both, however, have the typical appearance of intraepithelial squamous lesions of the lower female genital tract, and HPV changes are often evident (Fig. 19.6). Since no deep and irregular glandular clefts exist in the normal (non-adenosis-bearing) vagina, foci of high-grade VAIN accompanied by any extensions of carcinomatous epithelium into the vaginal stroma should be carefully scrutinized to exclude the presence of invasion.

PROGNOSIS AND TREATMENT

Topical estrogens may speed regeneration of the vaginal mucosa after radiation therapy but the effects of radiation therapy on the vaginal squamous mucosa may persist for years. Although ploidy studies suggest that postirradiation dysplasia patients with aneuploid lesions have a poorer long-term prognosis than do those patients with diploid or polyploid ones, the long term prognosis for both groups of patients is generally unclear.

Progression to invasive squamous cancer has been documented to occur roughly 1–4 years after treatment for high-grade VAIN. Excisional biopsy is probably adequate treatment for smaller lesions; however, larger and more extensive lesions may require partial or total vaginectomy. Other treatment modalities include cryosurgery, laser treatment, and intravaginal 5FU cream.

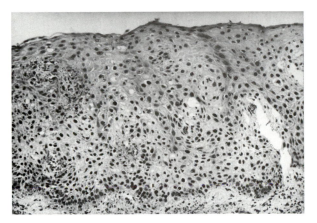

Figure 19.1. Radiation-induced vaginal squamous atypia.

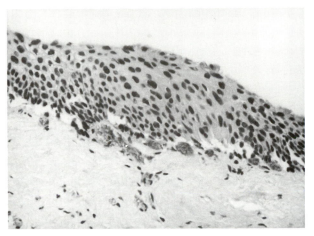

Figure 19.2. Radiation-induced vaginal squamous atypia.

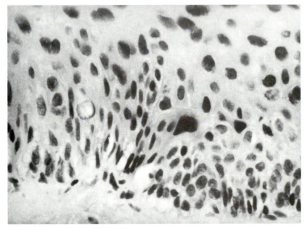

Figure 19.3. Radiation-induced vaginal squamous atypia.

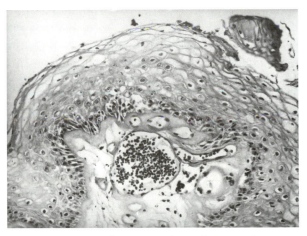

Figure 19.4. Radiation-induced vaginal mucosal changes.

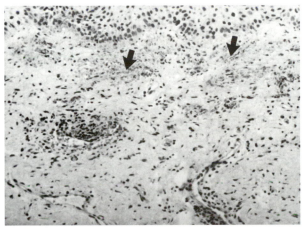

Figure 19.5. Radiation-induced vaginal mucosal changes.

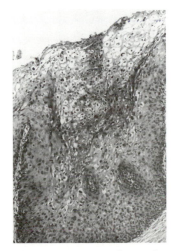

Figure 19.6. High grade vaginal intraepithelial neoplasia (VAIN).

20. Erosive Lichen Planus
vs.
Desquamative Inflammatory Vaginitis
vs.
Tampon-Related Genital Ulceration

CLINICAL

Vaginal ulcers are uncommon. Most have been regarded as due to infectious agents such as Herpes simplex, Treponema pallidum, and chlamydia; however, other etiologies include longstanding intravaginal foreign bodies such as diaphragms and pessaries, as well as certain toiletries.

The capacity for lichen planus (LP) to present as erosive and desquamative lesions of the oral mucosa, rarely in association with vulvar and vaginal lesions, is well described. Some regard desquamative inflammatory vaginitis (DIV) to be a form of erosive LP; however, since no consensus has been reached on this issue, DIV will be discussed as a separate, or perhaps closely related, disease. Clinically, DIV may mimic severe mucosal atrophy but in the face of normal estrogen levels. DIV affects women most often in their late reproductive to early menopausal phase, when adequate estrogen levels result from either endogenous means or as replacement therapy. Common complaints include vaginal irritation and soreness, burning, and dyspareunia with contact bleeding. Erosive or ulcerative oral lesions that accompany DIV may occur before or after the onset of the vulvovaginal ones, often by months or years. About a third of women with DIV give no history of concurrent or previous erosive or ulcerative oral lesions.

Tampon-related genital ulcerations (TRGUs) appear to be increasing in number and are most common in women in their mid-20s; indeed, tampons have been recognized as the most common cause of vaginal ulcers. The ulcers bleed on contact and cause vaginal spotting.

GROSS

The gross appearance of both erosive LP and DIV will be discussed together because of their similarities. Either all or a portion of the vaginal mucosa appears reddened, inflamed, and denuded, often covered by either a seropurulent exudate or a gray-tan pseudomembrane. The vulvar vestibule frequently appears eroded. If vaginal dilatation is not effected, adhesions begin to form in the upper vagina, eventually leading to obliteration. Oral exam on such patients may reveal a reticulated, gray lacy pattern, particularly in the buccal mucosa, that may also be present on the medial surfaces of the labia minora.

Vaginal TRGUs are usually present in the fornices, and most are >2cm in diameter, although microulcerations may occur. The edges of a TRGU are sharply demarcated and often rolled, with a clean red granulation tissue base. Colposcopic examination may reveal telltale evidence of cotton tampon fibers in the base of the ulcer (Fig. 20.1).

HISTOPATHOLOGY

The histopathologic features of ordinary LP are discussed in detail in Chapter 12. A vaginal biopsy from a patient with the typical clinical and gross appearance of DIV or erosive LP may be completely denuded of squamous epithelium (Fig. 20.2), exhibiting a relatively unremarkable-appearing ulcer; however, the surviving squamous mucosa elsewhere on the vulva may exhibit the characteristic changes of ordinary lichen planus (Fig. 20.3). The submucosa may exhibit immature granulation tissue infiltrated by dense acute and chronic inflammation sometimes covered by a thin layer of fibrin. The surrounding residual squamous mucosa may be thin with absence of maturation and disorganization of the basal and parabasal layers. The epithelium often shows cytoplasmic vacuolization.

The margins of the ulcer (Fig. 20.4) in vaginal TRGUs tend to be sharply demarcated from the edge of the surrounding squamous mucosa (Fig. 20.4—arrow), and the ulcer bed is quite clean. The adjacent squamous epithelium may show a separation between the intermediate and superficial layers; indeed, in some cases a cleft occurs between the basal layer and the overlying squamous epithelium, mimicking the appearance of pemphigus vulgaris. The ulcer base is composed of granulation tissue accompanied by neutrophils, lymphocytes, and plasma cells and a prominent vascular ectasia (Fig. 20.5).

In some cases, examination of the ulcer bed by polarized light will reveal the characteristic appearance of cotton fibers (Fig. 20.6) to support the diagnosis of TRGU.

PROGNOSIS AND TREATMENT

The mainstay of therapy for erosive LP has been topical and systemic corticosteroids. Some however, have advocated short courses of high-dose prednisone as well as retinoic acid derivatives as being effective treatment. However, the results have been far short of dramatic.

Spontaneous regressions are followed by severe exacerbations of disease. Remissions may take months to years to effect, and recurrences are common. Estrogen treatment appears to be ineffectual, and the vaginal walls become adherent to each other if proper dilatation is not maintained. Some patients with DIV have responded to clindamycin therapy but the treatment for it is currently controversial.

Discontinuation of tampon use for one or two menstrual cycles, allowing for spontaneous healing of the ulcers, is the treatment for vaginal TRGUs. Resumption of tampon use may cause recurrence of vaginal TRGUs.

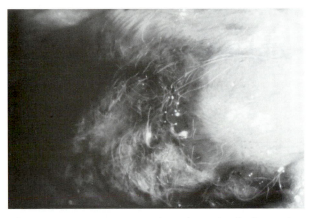

Figure 20.1. Tampon-related vaginal ulceration; cotton fibers in base of ulcer (high magnification colposcopic view).

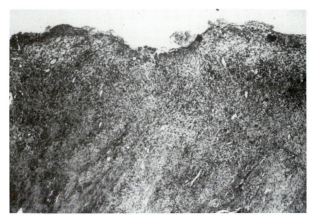

Figure 20.2. Desquamative inflammatory vaginitis.

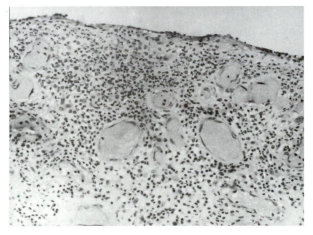

Figure 20.3. Erosive lichen planus-vagina.

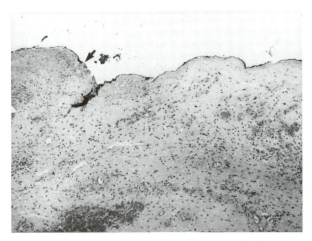

Figure 20.4. Tampon-related vaginal ulceration-edge of squamous mucosa at arrow.

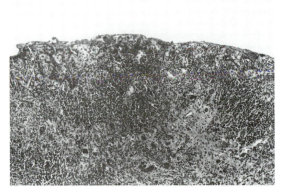

Figure 20.5. Tampon-related vaginal ulceration.

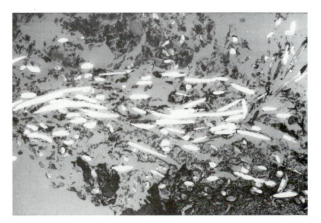

Figure 20.6. Tampon-related vaginal ulceration; polarized to show refractile cotton fibers in base of ulcer.

21. Vaginal Mucinous Adenosis

vs.

Vaginal Tuboendometrioid Adenosis

CLINICAL

Adenosis is defined as the presence of glandular epithelium or its mucinous products occurring in the vagina after completion of embryogenesis. Vaginal adenosis (VA) gained notoriety in the early 1970s after recognition of its association with intrauterine exposure to diethylstilbestrol (DES); the latter inhibits the upward growth of squamous epithelium from the urogenital sinus, leading to the retention of mullerian-derived glandular epithelium in the cervical portio and vagina. VA, however, is not a specific histologic marker for DES exposure. Both non-DES and DES-related VA are congenital and are usually asymptomatic.

GROSS

The gross and colposcopic appearance of VA depends largely on the age of the patient and the particular stage in the evolution of its "healing" by squamous metaplasia; prior to the latter, surface VA typically appears as granular to velvety erythematous patches reminiscent of the cervical eversion; the redness of the lesions may also impart the false appearance of mucosal ulceration. The areas of VA undergo "healing" through replacement by either maturing or immature squamous metaplasia; the latter appears as white epithelium that may show punctation or mosaicism.

VA and its resultant changes most commonly involve the upper third of the anterior vaginal wall and are restricted to the anterior vagina in slightly over half of the cases.

HISTOPATHOLOGY

In VA, the mucosa may exhibit either surface or stromal (lamina propria) involvement. The most commonly encountered combination (80% of cases) is both surface and stromal involvement by adenosis (Fig. 21.1); involvement of either surface or stroma alone is distinctly unusual. Three histologic types of VA are generally recognized: an embryonic type and the adult types, which include mucinous and so-called tuboendometrioid varieties. The embryonic type is more commonly seen in fetuses and stillborns but is rarely encountered in adults. It

occurs at the junction of the squamous epithelium and the stroma and consists of tiny glands with low cuboidal epithelium (Fig. 21.2), which may be easily overlooked. Approximately two-thirds of all cases of VA, including most of those that involve the mucosal surface (Fig. 21.1) and many of those with extension into the lamina propria (Fig. 21.1), are of the mucinous type. The glands of mucinous VA (Fig. 21.3) resemble those of the endocervix, as they are lined by tall columnar cells with abundant pale cytoplasm containing intracytoplasmic mucin. Not uncommonly, the mucinous surface epithelium has a papillary configuration (Figs. 21.1, 21.3). The tuboendometrioid (TEM) type is represented by ciliated glandular epithelium resembling the fallopian tube and/or the endometrium (Fig. 21.4); ultrastructural study of VA TEM glands reveal cells with typical cilia (Fig. 21.5). The TEM-type VA usually represents the glands in the lamina propria rather than on the surface. About one-fifth of cases of TEM adenosis are present in the upper vagina; although VA per se is rare in the lower vagina, when it does occur, it is more likely to be of the TEM type. The endocervical, or mucinous, variety of VA is more likely to give rise to the lesion that has been designated as microglandular hyperplasia (MGH). Similar to MGH occurring in the cervix (see Chapter 31), it typically exhibits a polypoid configuration and may appear worrisome because of its architectural features, which raise the question of a clear cell carcinoma. However, there is no significant nuclear atypicality, and mitotic figures are typically sparse to absent.

In areas where the adenotic glands are undergoing "healing," they are either partially (Fig. 21.6) or fully replaced by immature or mature squamous epithelium depending on the age of the patient. Because of replacement of adenotic glands in the lamina propria, there may be solid squamous nodules and rete pegs extending into the stroma similar to those observed in cervical squamous metaplasia. Extensive replacement of irregular adenotic glands by squamous metaplasia may simulate invasive squamous carcinoma. However, cytologic atypicality is absent, and the apparent islands of squamous cells show smooth, rounded contours, as opposed to the irregular outlines characteristic of invasive squamous cancer. Droplets of mucin, often without discernible mucinous glandular cells, are commonly encountered in such areas of squamous metaplasia.

PROGNOSIS AND TREATMENT

Malignant transformation occurs in 0.14–1.4 per 1000 DES-exposed women and probably even more rarely in those with congenital VA. Indeed, the vast majority of VA, particularly the mucosal surface glands, spontaneously "heal" through the process of squa-mous metaplasia (similar to that occurring in the cervi-cal transformation zone). Glands of VA deeper in the lamina propria may persist unchanged. Currently, there is no recommended treatment for biopsy-confirmed VA; however, patients are followed at least annually with a careful clinical examination and Pap smears.

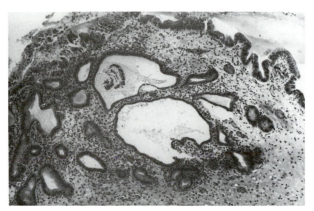

Figure 21.1. Vaginal tuboendometrioid-type adenosis-surface mucosal and stromal involvement.

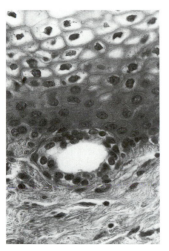

Figure 21.2. Vaginal adenosis-embryonic type.

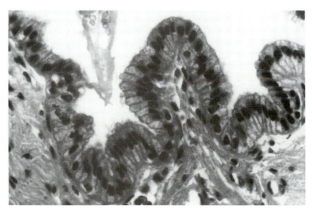

Figure 21.3. Vaginal adenosis-mucinous type.

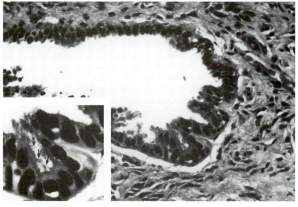

Figure 21.4. Vaginal adenosis-tuboendometrioid type (arrows-cilia).

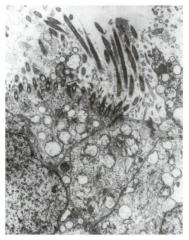

Figure 21.5. Electron micrograph of vaginal adenosis-tuboendometrioid type-showing ciliated epithelium.

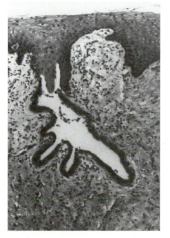

Figure 21.6. Vaginal surface and stromal adenosis showing partial replacement ("healing") by squamous metaplasia.

22. Atypical Vaginal Adenosis

vs.

Vaginal Clear Cell Carcinoma

CLINICAL

Compared to the usual (nonatypical) vaginal adenosis (VA) and vaginal clear cell carcinoma (CCC), relatively little information is available concerning so-called atypical VA. Some form of VA has been identified in 97% of patients with vaginal CCC and in 52% of patients with cervical CCC. However, atypical, or dysplastic, VA is uncommon; its maximum prevalence lies between 0.3% and 1.1% as detected by screening examinations and biopsy. Colposcopic examination has revealed areas of atypical VA to be flat but abnormally red secondary to a marked increase in normal-appearing blood vessels. Such an appearance contrasts with CCCs, most of which exhibit some degree of granularity, nodularity, or evidence of a mass effect.

Approximately two-thirds of women with CCC in the Registry for Research on Hormonal Transplacental Carcinogenesis (RRHTC) have a history of prenatal exposure to DES; 1 of 10 have a history of exposure to unidentified drugs, and 1 of 4 have a negative drug exposure history. Patients with CCC enrolled in the RRHTC range in age from 6 to 42 years, but the majority are between 17 and 21 (median age 19). In all cases DES was administered to mothers less than 18 weeks pregnant, and the total dose ranged within 300–18,000 mg. Complaints of abnormal vaginal bleeding and discharge have more often been accompanied larger tumors; however, up to one-fifth of CCC have been asymptomatic and detected only by digital palpation. Over half of CCC involve the vagina, usually the upper third of the anterior wall. Non-DES-associated lower-genital-tract CCCs have a bimodal distribution; about a third of patients are less than 25 years of age, and at least two-thirds of them are older than 45.

GROSS

As indicated earlier, to our knowledge, there appear to be no characteristic gross changes that permit the macroscopic identification of atypical VA.

Vaginal CCCs vary widely in size and ease of detection, ranging from microscopic size up to >10 cm in diameter. Indeed, rarely they may be virtually invisible to inspection with the naked eye or even with a colposcope if they are covered by normal and intact immature or mature squamous epithelium. Most CCCs, however, are relatively superficial and infiltrate only a few millimeters into the vaginal stroma. Those larger tumors may be nodular or assume a polypoid configuration, whereas others may exhibit flat features with ulceration and granularity as did this vaginal CCC from a 27-year-old woman with a history of DES exposure in utero (Fig. 22.1).

HISTOPATHOLOGY

Atypical VA virtually always occurs in the tuboendometrioid (TEM) type of glands, and there may be a spectrum of glandular atypicality among lesions. In some cases, low-power examination reveals only mild to moderate architectural atypia, manifested by TEM type glands with architectural complexity (Fig. 22.2) more complex and irregular than those of usual, or nonatypical, TEM. Although somewhat more crowded than typical TEM glands, they are more regular in their architectural configuration than CCC and lack the appearance of invasive cancer. At higher magnification, such glands of atypical TEM adenosis are lined by cells that have fairly abundant cytoplasm and mild to moderately pleomorphic nuclei (Fig. 22.3); they do not, however, possess the degree of atypicality characteristic of full-blown carcinoma. Nuclei are usually round to oval and may show considerable intraglandular variation in size and shape, some appearing more atypical than others (Fig. 22.3). Many of the nuclei contain prominent nucleoli. The cells may exhibit hobnail formation. Mitotic activity is rarely brisk; in fact, even 75% of full-blown CCC have a mitotic index of ≤1 per 10 high-power fields. DNA ploidy studies have been few but typical TEM adenosis is either euploid or polyploid, whereas atypical VA is often aneuploid. The atypical VA of TEM shown in Fig. 22.4 was found adjacent to a vaginal CCC; similar glands are frequently encountered in serially blocked vaginas at the periphery of overt CCC, engendering the speculation that atypical VA is a precursor lesion to that entity. Although cilia are not invariably present in atypical TEM adenosis, in some cases they may be easily identified, as shown in Figure 22.4 (arrows).

Other glands of mucinous-type atypical adenosis may show severe architectural abnormality on low-power examination, exhibiting an organoid configuration reminiscent of high-grade glandular atypia of the endocervix (Fig. 22.5). Higher magnification reveals marked glandular crowding, marked nuclear hyperchromasia and nuclear stratification, and brisk mitotic activity (Fig. 22.6).

CCC may exhibit three different growth patterns—tubulocystic, solid, and papillary—all of which may be seen in any of the female genital tract CCCs, especially the endometrium and the ovary. The most common is the tubulocystic pattern (Fig. 22.7) characterized by variable-sized glandular spaces that are lined by sometimes flattened and often bland-appearing low-cuboidal or columnar cells; the latter may assume a "hobnail" pattern with the cell apex bulging into the lumen (Fig. 22.8) and containing a prominent nucleus. The stromal cores of the supporting connective network may show impressive hyalinization (Fig. 22.8—arrows), a relatively common feature of any such CCC arising in the mullerian tract. Some CCCs of the vagina may have a striking similarity to the hypersecretory appearance of the Arias-Stella phenomenon within gestational endometrium, manifested by glands with intraglandular nuclear heterogeneity and hobnail-type cells with large, lobated nuclei (Fig. 22.9—arrow). Although mucin may be present in the lumens of CCC, it is seldom found in the cytoplasm. Papillary-type CCC exhibits epithelium similar to the tubulocystic variety but is found in a papillary configuration (Figs. 22.10, 22.11). The presence of psammoma bodies, occasionally in large numbers, may cause confusion with serous papillary carcinoma, either invading from the uterus or ovary, or primary in the vagina. Such a primary serous papillary carcinoma would be exceedingly rare in the vagina. Furthermore, the generally younger age group would also be distinctly unusual for a metastasis from the uterus or ovary. In the solid type of CCC, the cells are large and polygonal, with copious clear cytoplasm (Fig. 22.12); the latter is due to the presence of abundant intracytoplasmic glycogen that washes out in tissue processing and leaves a clear space. Occasional CCCs are arranged in cords of eosinophillic cells.

PROGNOSIS AND TREATMENT

Only one case of biopsied "endometrioid" VA in a DES-exposed woman has apparently progressed to adenocarcinoma. Despite the frequent finding of atypical VA at the periphery of serially sectioned vaginas of patients with CCC, there is currently no incontrovertible proof that atypical VA is a bona fide precursor to the cancer. Treatment of patients with atypical VA includes careful clinical follow-up with frequent meticulous examination, including colposcopic study and thorough digital palpation to exclude small submucosal nodules of CCC that are easily missed.

The major determinant of survival in patients with CCC is the stage of disease at diagnosis. Ninety percent of CCCs that present as stage I disease are restricted to the vagina, and have a 90% 5-year survival; stage II, III, and IV patients have 5 year survivals of 70, 30, and 20%, respectively. The overall actuarial 10-year survival is 79%. Patients <15 years of age appear to have a worse prognosis than do those age >19, and a tubulocystic microscopic pattern is associated with a more favorable prognosis; this may explain the better survival in those >19 since that pattern is 4 times more common in women in that age group.

Most recurrent CCCs involve the central pelvis and occur within 3 years of the primary diagnosis. The 5-year cumulative recurrence rate is about 25%, a poor prognostic factor since most of them died. Treatment of early-stage CCC usually includes radical hysterectomy, vaginectomy, and lymphadenectomy since there is a high rate of recurrence with only local excision. Radiotherapy probably is as effective as surgery in early-stage disease but is more commonly used in more advanced-stage tumors.

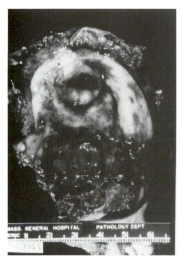

Figure 22.1. Vaginal clear cell carcinoma in an in utero DES-exposed young woman.

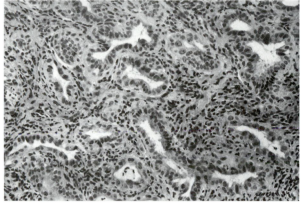

Figure 22.2. Atypical tuboendometrioid vaginal adenosis.

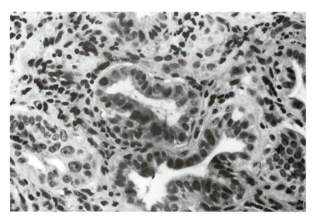

Figure 22.3. Atypical tuboendometrioid vaginal adenosis.

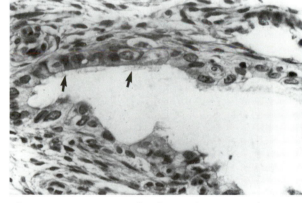

Figure 22.4. Atypical tuboendometrioid vaginal adenosis. Note prominent cilia (arrows).

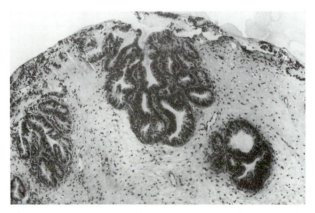

Figure 22.5. Atypical mucinous (endocervical-type) vaginal adenosis.

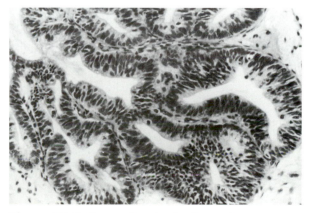

Figure 22.6. Severely atypical mucinous (endocervical-type) vaginal adenosis.

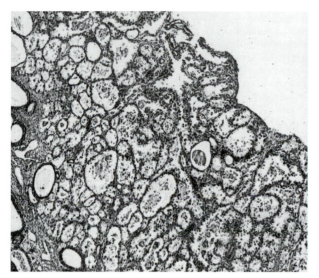

Figure 22.7. Vaginal clear cell carcinoma.

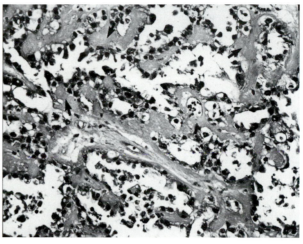

Figure 22.8. Vaginal clear cell carcinoma.

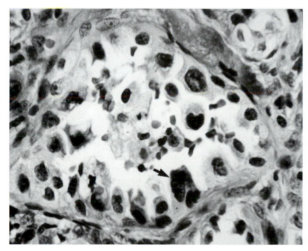

Figure 22.9. Vaginal clear cell carcinoma.

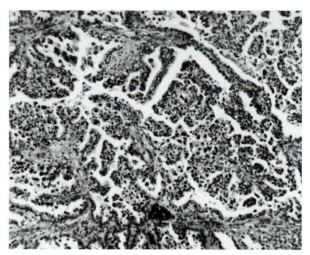

Figure 22.10. Vaginal clear cell carcinoma.

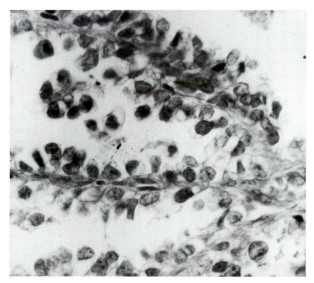

Figure 22.11. Vaginal clear cell carcinoma.

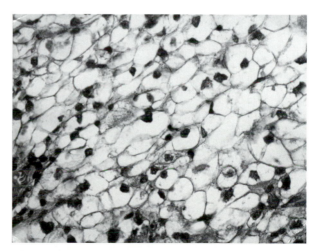

Figure 22.12. Vaginal clear cell carcinoma.

Section 3   CERVICAL DISORDERS

23. Cervical Intraepithelial Neoplasia (CIN): CIN 1 vs. CIN 2 vs. CIN 3; Squamous Intraepithelial Lesions (SIL): Low-Grade vs. High-Grade

CLINICAL

The prevalence of cervical intraepithelial neoplasia (CIN) has varied from 0.5 to 6.5% depending on the nature of the population screened. Over the past few decades, the prevalence of CIN has increased in teenagers and in women under the age of 30 years. Most women with CIN are asymptomatic or present with nonspecific symptoms such as vaginal discharge, pain, or local irritation. Anogenital HPV infection, presumably acquired through sexual contact, appears to assume most of the epidemiologic risk factors of CIN, including the number of lifetime sexual partners. Most studies indicate that there is a close correlation between histology and associated HPV type (especially in 16, 18, and 33) in CIN 2 and 3 and lack of correlation for CIN 1.

GROSS

CIN does not have a characteristic macroscopic appearance. The cervix usually appears normal, but occasionally shows nonspecific changes such as erosion, hyperemia, or leukoplakia. Areas affected with CIN usually fail to react with Iodine solution and remain as white or yellow in color (Schiller's test–positive). The test, however, cannot define the type of lesion present. The gross appearance of CIN is best appreciated by colposcopic examination after application of acetic acid. A variety of colposcopic patterns that reflect histopathologic changes of CIN and HPV infection in the epithelium include zones of white epithelium, foci showing a punctate vascular pattern, and mosaicism. When HPV infection is associated with multiple papillary fronds containing fibrovascular cores, the colposcopic findings are those of fine surface spikes. With experience, a rough correlation between the colposcopic appearance and the grade of CIN can be made. Most CIN lesions begin at the squamo-columnar junction of the transformation zone. Only about 10% of CIN involve the endocervical canal without involving the squamocolumnar junction. The size and endocervical extension of CIN tend to vary directly with increasing severity of grade.

HISTOLOGY

CIN is characterized by abnormalities in maturation, nuclear features, and mitotic activity. Abnormal maturation is manifested by loss of polarity and cellular disorganization. The degree of maturation is inversely related to the severity of the CIN. The nuclear abnormalities observed include enlargement, hyperchromasia, irregularity in size and shape, and chromatinic clumping. Nuclear abnormalities are very important criteria for the diagnosis of CIN and for determining its grade. The severity of the nuclear abnormality is inversely correlated with the amount of cellular differentiation. There is a rough correlation between the grade of CIN and the level at which mitotic figures and abnormal mitotic figures are found with increasing frequency in high-grade lesions. In addition, in approximately 20% of CIN lesions, abnormal differentiation in the form of hyperkeratosis, atypical parakeratosis, excess keratohyalin granules in the superficial layer and dyskeratosis are present.

CIN lesions are graded 1, 2, or 3 corresponding to mild, moderate, or severe dysplasia/carcinoma in situ, respectively. The CIN 1 category corresponds to low-grade squamous intraepithelial lesion (LSIL), and CIN 2 and 3 correspond to high-grade squamous intraepithelial lesion (HSIL) in The Bethesda System (TBS) for cytologic classification. This system does not necessarily require the reporting of the presence for HPV effect in either low-grade or high-grade lesions. In the future, this terminology may become applicable in histology because it provides uniformity of cytologic and histologic diagnosis and helps unify approach to patient management.

In CIN 1 (LSIL) abnormal proliferation of parabasal cells is confined to the lower third of the epithelium (Fig. 23.1). Although squamous maturation is maintained in the upper two-thirds of the epithelium, the cells at the surface still contain abnormal nuclei, which permits their detection in cytologic smears. The parabasal cells have increased nuclear cytoplasmic ratio. The nuclei in CIN 1 are relatively uniform in size and shape and are round or oval with a finely granular chromatin (Fig. 23.2). Mitotic activity is usually limited to the lower third of the epithelium.

CIN 2 and 3 (HSIL) constitute a morphologic continuum that merges with CIN 1. When the proliferation of atypical parabasal cells involves between one-third and two-thirds or more than two-thirds of the thickness of the epithelium, the lesion is classified as CIN 2 (Fig. 23.3) or 3, respectively. Nuclear abnormalities in CIN 2 are more marked than in CIN 1 and are manifested by a moderate degree of nuclear crowding and irregularities in nuclear size, nuclear shape, and chromatin pattern (Fig. 23.4). Mitotic figures, which may be abnormal, are present in the basal two-thirds of the epithelium, In CIN 3, almost the entire epithelium demonstrates high cellularity, immaturity, vertical orientation, and active proliferation (Fig. 23.5). Individual cells in CIN 3 are characterized by severe nuclear atypia in the form of hyperchromasia, irregularities of nuclear size and shape, and the presence of coarse chromatin (Fig. 23.6). Mitotic figures are present in all layers of the epithelium and may be numerous with many abnormal configurations.

It is now recognized that CIN 1 is the morphologic manifestation of productive HPV infection of the cervical squamous epithelium. The cytopathic effects of HPV infection include perinuclear cytoplasmic cavitation with thickening of the cytoplasmic membrane, nuclear atypia, and anisocytosis. These features have been termed *koilocytosis* or *koilocytotic atypia.* Episomal viral replication results in productive DNA synthesis with expression of the late viral genes, synthesis of structure proteins, and viral particles assembly in the superficial squamous epithelium. As such, koilocytosis manifests in the intermediate and superficial squamous cells and is more frequently present in CIN 1 lesions than CIN 2 or 3.

PROGNOSIS AND TREATMENT

The outcome for an individual lesion cannot be predicted with certainty. In general, CIN 1 (LSIL) is more likely to regress (more than half of cases) whereas the majority of CIN 2 and CIN 3 lesions (HSIL) persist on progress.

The management of CIN depends on the integration of the following procedures: cytology, colposcopy, direct cervical biopsy, endocervical curettage, and cervical cone biopsy. For CIN 1, if the entire lesion is visualized and the limits of the transformation zone are seen, the lesion can be excised or ablated, or the patient can be followed up carefully with no treatment. Excision or ablation should be considered for patients who are unlikely to return for follow-up or who strongly desire this therapy. Women with CIN 2 or 3 usually undergo colposcopy and directed biopsy. Following biopsy confirmation and delineation of the distribution of the lesion, excisional or ablative therapy aimed at removal or destruction of the entire lesion and transformation zone is usually performed in a nonpregnant woman.

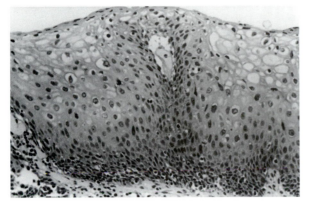

Figure 23.1. Cervical intraepithelial neoplasia 1. Human papilloma virus cytopathic effect is present in the upper layers.

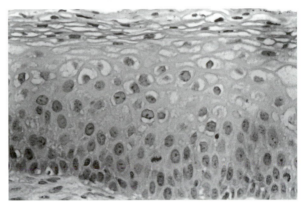

Figure 23.2. Cervical intraepithelial neoplasia 1. Abnormal cells are present in lower third.

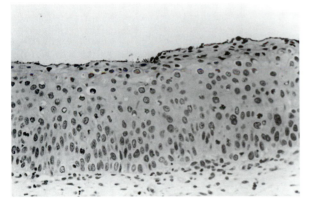

Figure 23.3. Cervical intraepithelial neoplasia 2. Mitotic figures are present in middle layer.

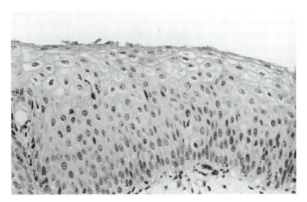

Figure 23.4. Cervical intraepithelial neoplasia 2.

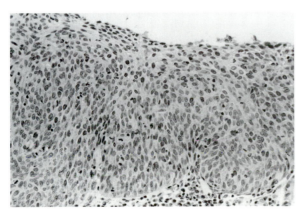

Figure 23.5. Cervical intraepithelial neoplasia 3. Full thickness loss of maturation.

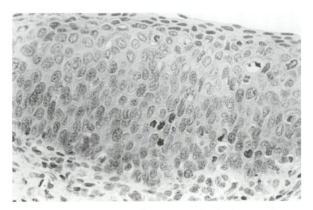

Figure 23.6. Cervical intraepithelial neoplasia 3.

24. Squamous Atrophy vs. Transitional Metaplasia vs. CIN

CLINICAL

CIN characteristically occurs in young women and those in the reproductive age group, and is uncommon in postmenopausal patients. The menopause is associated with diminished estrogenic stimulation of the squamous epithelium, which undergoes atrophy. Transitional metaplasia occurs predominantly, but not exclusively, on the ectocervix and is often associated with atrophy. Transitional metaplasia, however, has also been encountered in the transformation zone of perimenopausal and postmenopausal women.

HISTOLOGY

Atrophic epithelium shows marked decrease in thickness with lack or flattening of retepegs, loss of glycogen in intermediate cell layers, and little or no differentiation or maturation of the surface epithelium (Fig. 24.1). Atrophic epithelium may be composed entirely of a population of immature basal and parabasal cells (Fig. 24.2). These cells show high nucleus : cytoplasm ratios and have round or oval nuclei and occasional nucleoli.

Unlike CIN, atrophic epithelium lacks nuclear atypia and pleomorphism and mitotic activity is absent. In addition, cellular cohesion is normal and cytologic atypia are absent in the atrophic epithelium. There is no cellular disorganization or lack of polarity, which are characteristic of CIN. In older women, in whom it may occasionally be difficult to distinguish severe atrophy from high-grade CIN, a repeat biopsy after a course of topical estrogen cream often resolves the problem by inducing maturation in atrophic epithelium. In contrast, estrogen administration does not alter the appearance of CIN.

Transitional metaplasia is characterized by the presence of relatively monotonous elongated to ovoid transitional-type basal and parabasal cells occupying full thickness of the epithelium (Fig. 24.3). These cells typically have high nucleus : cytoplasm ratio and ovoid nuclei that display longitudinal nuclear grooves. The latter feature heightens the resemblance to transitional epithelium. This metaplasia, however, does not represent true urothelium, which has superficial maturation and terminal differentiation, leading to the characteristic layer of "umbrella" cells.

Transitional metaplasia can also be confused with high-grade CIN because the nuclei are crowded and the nucleus : cytoplasmic ratio is high (Figs. 24.4, 24.5). The lack of cytologic atypia, cellular disorganization and the palisaded appearance of the basal cell layer, as well as the low or absent mitotic activity, distinguish transitional metaplasia from high-grade CIN (Fig. 24.6). The nuclei in transitional metaplasia are also bland and may demonstrate uniform longitudinal grooves (Fig. 24.5).

The rare cases of inverted transitional cell papilloma and transitional cell carcinomas of the cervix may possibly have origin from foci to transitional metaplasia. The occurrence of these neoplasms in the cervix further illustrates the capability of the cervical epithelium to differentiate along urothelial cell lines.

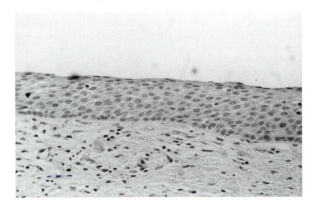

Figure 24.1. Atrophic squamous epithelium.

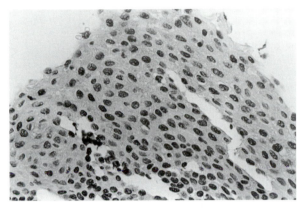

Figure 24.2. Atrophic squamous mucosa identified in an ECC from a 75 Year old woman.

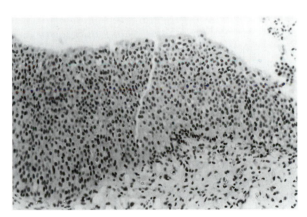

Figure 24.3. Transitional metaplasia.

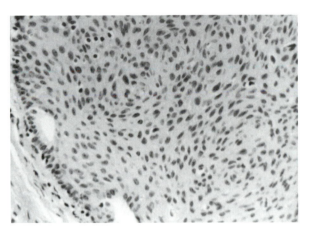

Figure 24.4. Transitional metaplasia.

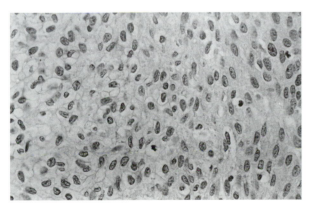

Figure 24.5. Transitional metaplasia. Bland oval nuclei with occasional grooves.

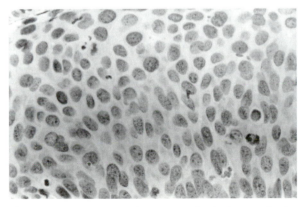

Figure 24.6. Cervical intraepithelial neoplasia 3.

25. Inflammatory Reactive Atypia

vs.

CIN

CLINICAL

Acute and chronic cervicitis may be related to infectious or noninfectious etiologies. The former may be caused by a variety of organisms such as *Trichomonas, Candida, Hemophilus vaginalis, Chlamydia,* and *Neisseria gonorrhoea,* and, less commonly, viral or granulomatous diseases. The latter may be related to chemical irritation, or iatrogenic causes such as previous surgical procedures. The causative organism or agent, however, may be unknown. In cases of acute or longstanding inflammation or infection, the squamous epithelium undergoes reactive and reparative changes. These changes have been variably designated as squamous atypia or inflammatory atypia and have been reported in approximately 2–3% of all cervical smears. It encompasses a heterogeneous group of lesions, some of which may also represent the earliest, but nonspecific, cellular manifestations of HPV infection.

HISTOLOGY

Cervicitis may be characterized by the presence of mucosal denudation, inflammatory reactive epithelial atypia, and mixed inflammatory infiltrate. Lymphoid follicles may also be present, prompting the diagnosis of follicular cervicitis.

The "atypical" squamous epithelium may be slightly thickened with diminished intracellular glycogen (Figs. 25.1, 25.2, 25.3). Hyperkeratosis may be observed. The squamous cells are uniform, and there is retention of overall cellular organization, polarity, and an orderly pattern of maturation. The atypical basal cells occupy the lower one-third of the epithelium, and there is minimal mitotic activity (Fig. 25.3). The cells have distinct cell membranes and retain a relatively normal nucleus : cytoplasm ratio. The nuclei have smooth, round, and regular nuclear outline, with finely granular and equally distributed chromatin. They contain prominent chromocenters and nucleoli. Epithelial cells above the enlarged basal zones display normal maturation. Typically, there is an associated dense, acute or chronic inflammatory infiltrate that involves the epithelium and the underlying stroma.

Inflammatory/reparative atypia may be characterized by considerable cellular alterations of the squamous epithelium, which should not be misinterpreted as CIN (Fig. 25.4). In contrast to squamous atypia, CIN shows cellular crowding and disorganization with loss of normal squamous maturation, the severity of which depends on the grade of the CIN (Fig. 25.5). The nuclei in CIN show pleomorphism, nuclear wrinkling, and hyperchromasia, and mitotic figures, often abnormal, may be prominent (Fig. 25.6).

In summary, reactive and reparative process differ from CIN in that repair shows severe inflammation, rare mitosis, large uniform nuclei, finely powdered chromatin and macronucleoli. CIN on the other hand is rarely severely inflamed, shows numerous mitosis and demonstrates nuclear pleomorphism with clumping of chromatin, and nucleoli are usually small or absent.

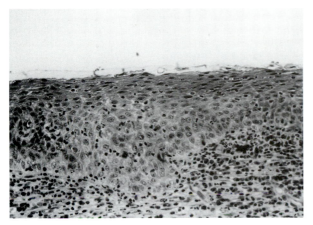

Figure 25.1. Squamous epithelium with reparative changes.

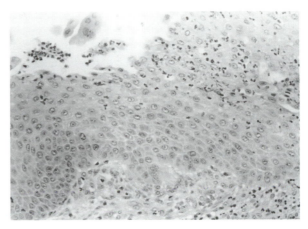

Figure 25.2. Squamous epithelium reparative changes.

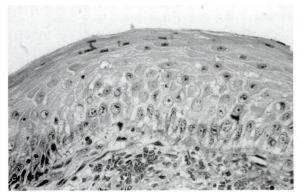

Figure 25.3. Repair characterized by large cells in lower third with open chromatin and nucleoli.

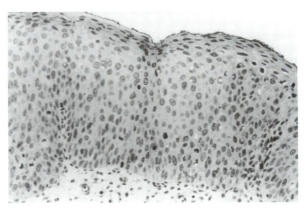

Figure 25.4. Cervical intraepithelial neoplasia 2.

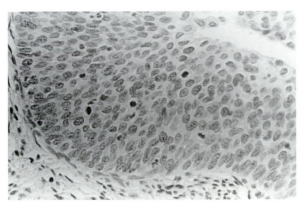

Figure 25.5. Cervical intraepithelial neoplasia 3.

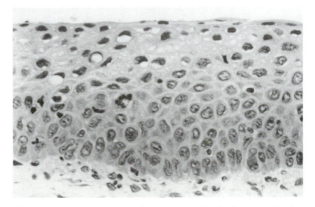

Figure 25.6. Cervical intraepithelial neoplasia 2. Nuclear overlapping, loss of polarity and hyperchromasia.

26. Reserve Cell Hyperplasia

vs.

Atypical Immature Metaplasia

vs.

CIN

CLINICAL

Reserve cell hyperplasia and immature squamous cell metaplasia represent early stages of maturation in which increasing differentiation gradually results in mature squamous metaplasia. It is a frequently occurring nonspecific reaction of the endocervical mucosa that is often found in pregnant women, women using oral contraceptives, and postmenopausal women.

HISTOLOGY

Reserve cell hyperplasia is defined as the appearance of one or more layers of primitive undifferentiated cell beneath the columnar lining epithelium of the endocervix and the underlying basement membrane (Fig. 26.1). Reserve cells are cuboidal to low columnar with round to oval nuclei and scant cytoplasm. This nonspecific reaction of the endocervical mucosa is usually observed proximal to the site of immature squamous metaplasia. The acid pH of the vagina, chronic infection, and prolonged irritation are some of the stimuli that cause the metaplastic change in the everted endocervical epithelium.

Immature squamous metaplasia represents the morphologic spectrum of epithelial differentiation as the single layer or multiple layers of reserve cells acquire more abundant eosinophilic cytoplasm and features of mature nonkeratinizing epithelial cells (Fig. 26.2). The nuclei are uniform with smooth nuclear membranes, finely granular chromatin, and prominent nucleoli. Mitotic figures may be abundant, sometimes even close to the surface. A layer of mucinous epithelium on the surface representing the last remnant of endocervical epithelium that is replaced by the metaplastic squamous epithelium may be present (Fig. 26.3). The most helpful features in distinguishing CIN 2 and 3 from immature squamous metaplasia are the retention of cell polarity, lack of crowding, and absence of nuclear pleomorphism in the latter (Figs. 26.4, 26.5, 26.6). Abnormal mitotic figures are not present in immature squamous metaplasia. The chromatin is finer and more evenly distributed than in high-grade CIN. Mucinous epithelium often is present on the surface of the immature metaplastic squamous epithelium and rarely overlies CIN.

Occasionally, slight nuclear enlargement and atypia may be observed in immature metaplasia, and such lesions may be designated by some as *atypical immature metaplasia*. This term, however, is not widely accepted and may be confusing to clinicians. The "atypical cells" in this lesion usually occupy the lower two-thirds of the epithelium and are often vertically arranged. Although this lesion may be difficult to distinguish it from CIN 2 or 3, cell polarity is retained, cell membranes are clearly defined, and the nuclei of atypical immature metaplasia are only slightly enlarged and round, with finely granular chromatin. The prominent cellular crowding, disorganization, pleomorphism, hyperchromasia, and abnormal mitotic figures observed in CIN are not present in atypical immature squamous metaplasia.

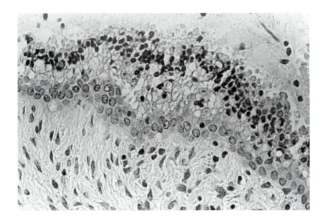

Figure 26.1. Reserve cell hyperplasia.

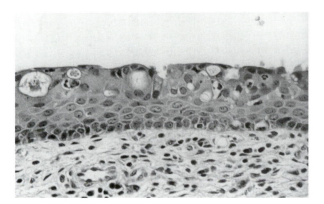

Figure 26.2. Immature squamous metaplasia.

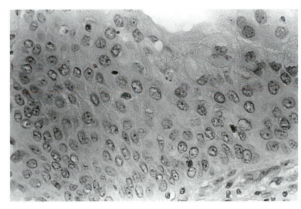

Figure 26.3. Immature squamous metaplasia.

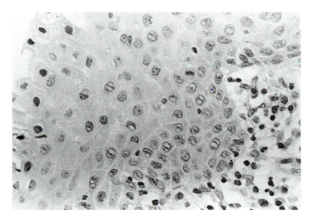

Figure 26.4. Immature squamous metaplasia.

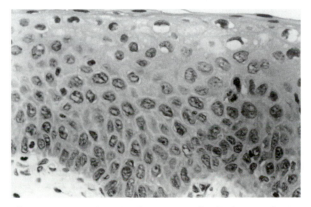

Figure 26.5. Cervical intraepithelial neoplasia 2.

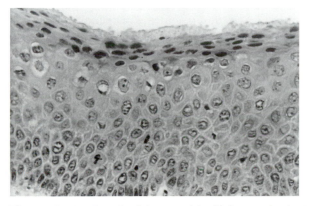

Figure 26.6. Cervical intraepithelial neoplasia 3 with surface parakeratosis.

27. Koilocytosis

vs.

Koilocytotic-like changes

vs.

Normal Glycogenated Epithelium

HISTOLOGY

Koilocytotic change, which is the histologic hallmark of HPV infection, is usually found in squamous epithelium in which the cellular architecture is disorganized and maturation is abnormal (Fig. 27.1). There is usually some degree of proliferation in the parabasal layer. The cell membranes of koilocytotic cells are thickened, and the nucleus is often eccentric with a distinct, clear perinuclear halo (Fig. 27.2). The nucleus shows variable degrees of anisonucleosis, hyperchromasia, heterochromasia, wrinkling, and irregularities of the nuclear membrane. Binucleation is common.

Perinuclear clearings may also occur as a reflection of atrophy/inflammatory-related vacuolar degeneration in non-HPV-related infections, notably *Trichomonas vaginalis, G. vaginalis,* and *candidiasis* (Fig. 27.3). The associated reactive squamous atypia may show, in addition to the perinuclear halos in the intermediate and superficial cells, rounding of the nuclei with slight coarsening of chromatin pattern (Fig. 27.4). Unlike koilocytes, however, the perinuclear halo associated with non-HPV infections is not sharply demarcated, and the nuclei are not enlarged. Nuclear wrinkling and hyperchromasia are absent. Normal stratification and maturation are maintained, and there is no proliferation in the parabasal layers (Fig. 27.4). In contrast, koilocytotic epithelium always manifests some degree of disorganization, particularly near the surface, and there is a disturbance in the normal pattern of maturation. The nuclei in reactive changes remain centrally located, and there is no evidence of significant nuclear atypia (Fig. 27.4). The cell borders are not accentuated or thickened.

In cases where the differential diagnosis between koilocytosis and koilocytotic-like changes associated with other infectious remains difficult, a descriptive diagnosis may be appropriate. These cases may show cytoplasmic halos with very mild nuclear atypia in the absence of binucleate cells or binucleate cells in the context of epithelial architecture typical or metaplastic or reactive process.

Koilocytotic-like changes, including nuclear enlargement, hyperchromasia, and cytoplasmic halos, may also be observed in postmenopausal epithelium unrelated to HPV. This change has been designated by some as postmenopausal squamous atypia or "pseudokoilocytosis." These postmenopausal "atypias" show more uniformity in size and contours of the perinuclear halos, lesser nuclear enlargement (usually ≤ 2-fold), milder nuclear staining intensity, and a more finely and/or evenly distributed nuclear chromatin than HPV-associated LSIL lesions.

Metaplastic squamous epithelium with prominent cytoplasmic vacuolization may also be confused with koilocytotic change (Fig. 27.5). The cells of metaplastic squamous epithelium have a perinuclear clearing that is not sharply demarcated, and the nuclei are not enlarged or atypical. Binucleation and nuclear atypia, including anisokaryosis, pleomorphism, and polychromasia, are also the hallmarks of HPV-related process and are absent in metaplastic squamous epithelium (Fig. 27.6).

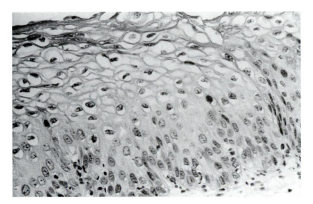

Figure 27.1. Cervical intraepithelial neoplasia 1 with prominent koilocytotic change.

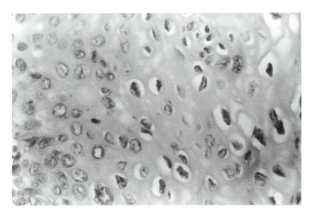

Figure 27.2. Koilocytotic cells.

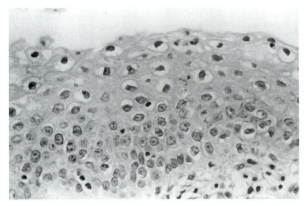

Figure 27.3. Koilocytotic-like change associated with inflammation.

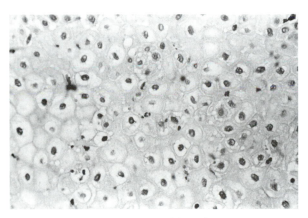

Figure 27.4. Koilocytotic-like change.

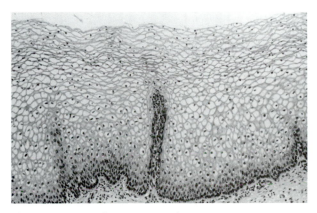

Figure 27.5. Glycogenated squamous epithelium.

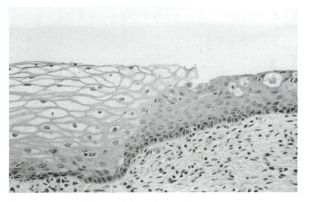

figure 27.6. Transition from immature squamous metaplasia to glycogenated metaplastic epithelium.

28. Endocervical Cleft Involvement by CIN

vs.

Superficial Invasive (Microinvasive) Squamous Cell Carcinoma

CLINICAL

Most patients with superficial invasive (microinvasive) squamous carcinoma are asymptomatic and the lesion is detected initially in cytologic smears and confirmed subsequently by punch biopsies, conization, or hysterectomy specimens. The incidence of superficial invasive carcinoma is estimated at 5–10% of specimens excised for in situ squamous carcinoma, 8–10% of invasive squamous cancers, and 12% of clinical stage 1 cervical cancer. The mean age of this group of patients, 38.2 years, has varied over the years because of changes in the definition of microinvasion and increasing use of cytology screening, which has reduced the frequency of frankly invasive carcinoma.

The clinical features of patients with endocervical cleft involvement by CIN are those discussed earlier for CIN.

GROSS

In superficial invasive squamous carcinoma, the cervix is usually grossly normal or demonstrates nonspecific findings, such as chronic cervicitis or erosion. The gross appearance of superficial invasive carcinoma, similar to that in CIN lesions, is best appreciated on colposcopic examination. A variety of colposcopic patterns may be seen, but the presence of abnormal vessels is considered to be the most characteristic.

HISTOLOGY

Extension of CIN into underlying endocervical clefts, is generally directly related to the severity of CIN. This histopathologic picture can mimic microinvasion, especially if the gland involvement is tangentially sectioned. The presence of residual glandular epithelium often facilitates the diagnosis. These foci also typically have the smooth configuration of bulky rete pegs or expanded, round, well-circumscribed nests of typical squamous epithelium (Fig. 28.1). Loss of cell polarity and nuclear palisade characteristic of invasion are absent. The basement membranes remain intact and there is usually no surrounding desmoplastic stromal response (28.2, 28.3). Serially sectioning through the tissue can usually demonstrate the continuity of the extension of the CIN lesion from the surface epithelium into underlying endocervical clefts. The nidus of well-differentiated cells originating from the basal layer of the epithelium, confluence of tumor nests, and lymphatic/vascular space invasion that are features of microinvasion, are absent in CIN extension into endocervical glands. The presence of central necrosis within an intraglandular CIN3 lesion, however, should alert the pathologist to look for invasion.

A definitive diagnosis of superficial invasive carcinoma is made on histologic evaluation of cervical tissue removed by conization or hysterectomy. Microinvasive squamous cell carcinoma is most commonly associated with extensive CIN 3 involving either the surface of the cervix or the endocervical crypts (Fig. 28.4). Much less commonly, the overlying epithelium resembles CIN 2, or rarely, CIN 1. The FIGO has defined stage 1A tumors as those invasive cancers identified only microscopically. The invasion should be limited to measured stromal invasion with a maximum depth of 5.0 mm and no wider than 7.0 mm. The depth of invasion should be measured from the base of the epithelium, either surface or glandular, from which it originates. Vascular space involvement, either venous or lymphatic, does not alter the staging. In stage $1A_1$ lesions, the measured invasion of stroma should not exceed 3.0 mm in depth and no wider than 7.0 mm. Stage $1A_2$ tumors have a measured invasion of stroma >3 mm but <5 mm and ≤7 mm. All clinical and gross lesions even with a superficial invasion but confined to cervix are designated as stage 1B.

The histopathologic features associated with early invasion include loss of nuclear palisade, cellular enlargement, and maturation at the stromal–epithelial interface, angulation and scalloping of the epithelial borders, and desmoplastic stromal response. In the earliest invasion, a nidus of well-differentiated cells with more abundant eosinophilic cytoplasm and more prominent nucleoli adjacent to noninvasive cells forms at the base of an intraepithelial lesion (Fig. 28.5). This focus expands to form a tongue-like process projecting into the underlying stroma. The most common progression of cellular growth patterns of neoplastic cells in the stroma are finger-like processes or networks of confluent strands, and infrequently small isolated nests or clusters (Fig. 28.6). The presence of a nidus of well-differentiated cells or keratinization in the background on an intraepithelial lesion should stimulate the search for areas of incipient invasion, and multiple serial cuts should be requested.

Invasion incites a variety of stromal responses, including chronic inflammation, a desmoplastic reaction, occasional formation of granulomas around necrotic cells or keratin debris, and dilation of capillary/lymphatic spaces. Capillary/lymphatic space invasion may be present and should be recognized only when these spaces are lined by clearly recognizable endothelial cells.

PROGNOSIS AND TREATMENT

The prognosis and management of microinvasive squamous cell carcinoma is generally dependent on the depth and pattern of invasion, presence, or absence of lymphovascular space involvement, tumor volume and horizontal extent, and the status of the surgical margins. Patients with microinvasive carcinoma who are desirous of maintaining fertility may be managed with conization provided they undergo careful, periodic follow-up and clearly understand that there is measurable risk of developing pelvic lymph node metastases or recurrent disease. In this subgroup of patients, there is low incidence of nodal involvement (0.7%). When the depth of invasion increases to 3–5 mm, the risk of nodal involvement increases (4.3%). At most centers, the recommended therapy for microinvasive carcinoma that fulfills FIGO stage 1A is a simple hysterectomy. The status of the cone margins are also important factors as patients with positive margins for CIN are much more likely to have residual invasive carcinoma in hysterectomy specimens than are women with negative margins.

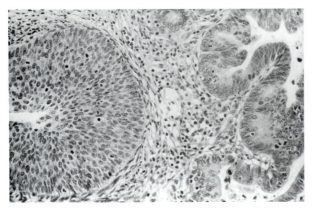

Figure 28.1. Cervical intraepithelial neoplasia 3 involving endocervical gland (left side). Adenocarcinoma in situ of endocervical epithelium is also present(right side).

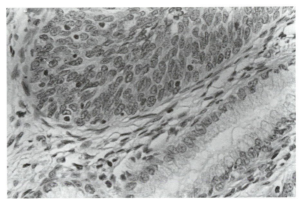

Figure 28.2. Cervical intraepithelial neoplasia 3 involving endocervical glands.

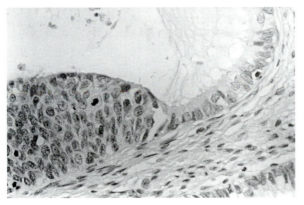

Figure 28.3. Cervical intraepithelial neoplasia 3 involving endocervical gland.

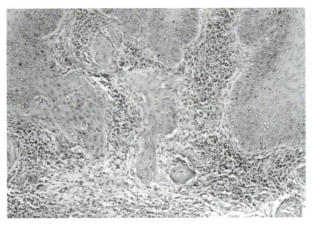

Figure 28.4. Microinvasive squamous cell carcinoma.

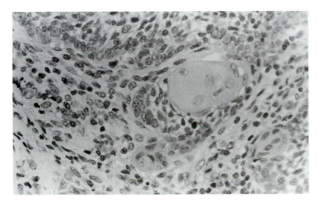

Figure 28.5. Squamous differentiation in microinvasive carcinoma.

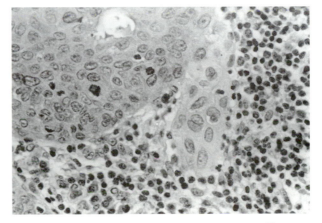

Figure 28.6. Microinvasive squamous cell carcinoma.

29. Poorly Differentiated Squamous Cell Carcinoma

vs.

Glassy Cell Carcinoma

CLINICAL

Glassy cell carcinoma is rare and represents less than 2% of all cervical carcinoma. It has been generally considered to be the least differentiated form of adenosquamous cell carcinoma and accounts for 20% of tumors in that category. Glassy cell carcinoma occurs in patients who are somewhat younger (mean age 31–41 years) than patients with conventional squamous cell or adenocarcinoma of the cervix. Despite the initially unexpected number of cases manifesting an association between pregnancy and glassy cell carcinoma, more recent reports have shown that this association is weak. Presenting symptoms are usually vaginal bleeding and discharge.

Most patients with squamous cell carcinoma are between the ages of 45 and 55 years of age at the time of diagnosis. Recently, however, there has been increasing realization that cervical cancer can occur in patients under 35 years of age. The majority of patients present with abnormal vaginal bleeding. With progression of disease, vaginal discharge and pain may be evident. Some patients with stage I disease, however, are frequently asymptomatic, and the lesion is detected on the basis of an abnormal PAP smear.

GROSS

Glassy cell carcinoma usually presents as a bulky exophytic mass. It may also diffusely infiltrate the cervix to form a barrel-shaped cervix. Characteristically, however, there is less deep invasion than suspected from the size of the protuberant mass.

Invasive squamous cell carcinoma displays a wide range of gross appearances. The lesions may be exophytic, polypoid, papillary, infiltrative, or ulcerative. The surface is usually granular, and the areas bleed readily on touch. Large tumors may produce a barrel-shaped cervix, while endophytic lesions that extensively invade the stroma result in a firm lesion with minimal surface change. The majority of early carcinomas are localized within the transformation zone. Colposcopic examination usually reveals atypical tortuous vessels varying widely in size and configuration over a slightly elevated and granular area.

HISTOLOGY

Glassy cell carcinoma is characterized by the presence of nests and solid sheets of cells often separated by delicate fibrous stroma (Fig. 29.1). The fibrous stroma typically contains a prominent inflammatory infiltrate composed predominantly of eosinophils and plasma cells. The neoplastic cells are large and polygonal, and have distinct cell borders that can be highlighted with a PAS stain. The cytoplasm is moderate to abundant in amount and is characteristically finely granular or ground-glass and stains eosinophilic or amphophilic (Fig. 29.2). The cells contain uniformly large round to oval nuclei, with prominent single or multiple nucleoli (Fig. 29.3). Mitotic figures are numerous. The tumor does not show apparent squamous nor glandular differentiation. Occasionally, minor degrees of individual cell keratinization, infrequent intercellular bridges, and rare aborted lumens and intracellular mucin positivity, however, may be noted, but usually these areas are focal and inconspicuous. The overlying surface squamous epithelium may be normal or may show CIN.

Poorly differentiated squamous cell carcinoma is composed of masses and nests of immature cells with scant cytoplasm, marked nuclear pleomorphism, and high mitotic activity (Fig. 29.4). The cells have scant indistinct cytoplasm, have hyperchromatic oval or spindle-shaped nuclei, and resemble the cells in high-grade CIN (Fig. 29.5). Keratinization is minimal or absent. Poorly differentiated squamous cell carcinomas occasionally are composed of large bizarre and highly pleomorphic cells with giant, bizarre nuclei and numerous abnormal mitotic figures.

Unlike glassy cell carcinoma, large cell nonkeratinizing squamous cell carcinoma generally lacks the ground-glass appearance of the cytoplasm of the cell, seldom exhibits prominent nucleoli, and shows more than a minor degree of squamous differentiation. The chromatin of cells of nonkeratinizing squamous cell carcinoma also is coarser and distributed along the nuclear membrane (Fig. 29.6).

Although the classic description of glassy cell carcinoma implies an undifferentiated mixed adenosquamous carcinoma, many of the poorly differentiated large cell nonkeratinizing squamous cell carcinoma project a histologic picture almost identical to that of glassy cell carcinoma. In addition, poor fixation and pale staining of paraffin sections tend to obscure the features of nonkeratinizing squamous cell carcinoma to the degree that it may resemble glassy cell. Recent studies have demonstrated that these large cell nonkeratinizing squamous cell carcinoma with some features of glassy cell were found to have a prognosis similar to that for glassy cell carcinoma. The restrictive diagnosis of glassy cell carcinoma should be applied to tumors composed virtually or exclusively of large cells with conspicuous eosinophilic amphophilic cytoplasm that have a ground-glass appearance.

PROGNOSIS AND TREATMENT

In general, glassy cell carcinomas have been shown to have an aggressive clinical course with a high frequency of pelvic and extrapelvic spread and poor response to surgery and/or radiotherapy. Addition of adjuvant chemotherapy for the management of these patients has been suggested. The 5-year survival rate for glassy cell carcinoma is in the range of 31–33%, which is lower than that of survival of squamous cell carcinoma (50%). Some studies, however, did not demonstrate a significantly different course as compared to nonkeratinizing squamous cell carcinoma for the same stage.

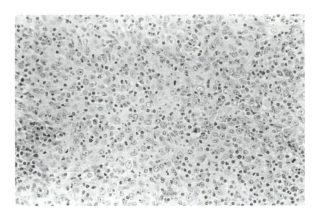

Figure 29.1. Glassy cell carcinoma.

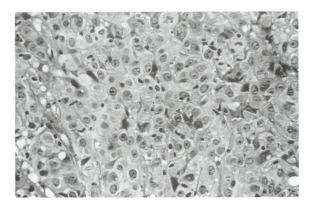

Figure 29.2. Glassy cell carcinoma.

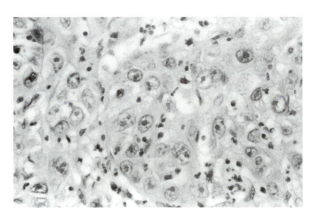

Figure 29.3. Glassy cell carcinoma.

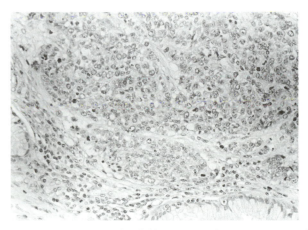

Figure 29.4. Poorly differentiated squamous cell carinoma, large cell nonkeratinizing type.

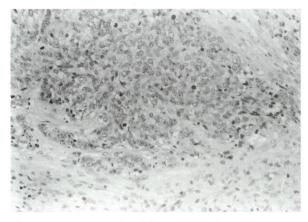

Figure 29.5. Poorly differentiated squamous cell carcinoma, large cell nonkeratinizing type.

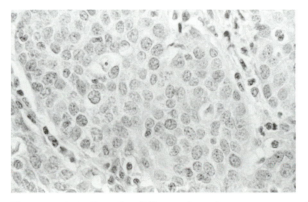

Figure 29.6. Poorly differentiated squamous cell carcinoma, large cell nonkeratinizing type.

30. Cervical Decidual Reaction
vs.
Placental Site Nodule
vs.
Large Cell Nonkeratinizing Squamous Cell Carcinoma

CLINICAL

Decidual transformation of the cervical stroma may occur during pregnancy or in patients treated with progestins. It has been estimated that approximately one-third of cervical biopsy specimens or hysterectomy specimens at full term show a cervical decidual reaction. This reaction typically disappears at ~8 weeks postpartum.

Patients with placental site nodule are usually in the reproductive age group ranging from 20 to 47 years with a mean age of 31 years. All have successfully completed at least one pregnancy. The mean period since last documented pregnancy is 29 months. Placental site nodule may represent a portion of the implantation site that persists after the last pregnancy and is unlikely to represent an implantation site of a more recent clinically unrecognized pregnancy. They are usually discovered incidentally in biopsies, usually endometrial; and less commonly in endocervical curettage, performed for a number of unrelated gynecologic problems such as menorrhagia or infertility, or for evaluation of CIN. Occasionally the diagnosis is made as an incidental finding on a hysterectomy specimen, but more commonly a hysterectomy that was performed subsequent to rendering the diagnosis on curettage may reveal residual lesion and help in establishing the diagnosis.

The clinical features of large cell nonkeratinizing squamous cell carcinoma are presented in Chapter 29.

GROSS

Decidual reaction of the cervical stroma frequently presents as raised yellowish or red streaks, discrete nodules, or pseudopolyps. These lesions are usually soft and friable and bleed easily following trauma. Rarely a fulminant decidual reaction may transform into fungating masses that may be colposcopically mistaken for invasive carcinoma.

Placental site nodules are usually incidental findings located in the endometrium above the lower uterine segment. These nodules may, however, be found in the lower uterine segment and in the upper endocervix in one-third of cases. In a few cases the placental site nodules were totally devoid of surrounding tissue, precluding accurate assessment of location. All the placental site nodules are usually microscopic in size and only rarely grossly visible. The latter may be noted in some of the hysterectomy specimens as a small, firm, yellow excrescence in the endometrium; as a pale tan nodule in the superficial myometrium; or as a hemorrhagic nodule just above the internal os. One reported example had arisen within the cervix as a polypoid endocervical mass.

The gross features of large cell nonkeratinizing squamous cell carcinoma are presented in Chapter 29.

HISTOLOGY

Cervical decidual reactions may present just beneath the epithelium or as an endocervical polypoid protrusion composed largely of decidual cells. The overlying superficial epithelium is usually extremely thin and may be partially eroded. Decidualized cells are large, with abundant eosinophilic pale granular cytoplasm and well-defined cytoplasmic membranes (Figs. 30.1, 30.2). Their nuclei are usually round and bland with conspicuous nucleoli. If degenerative changes occur, these cells may be irregular, with hyperchromatic nucleoli. These cells are identical to gestational decidual cells of endometrium. Focal collections of lymphocytes and occasionally polymorphonuclear (leukocytes) may be pronounced surrounding the decidua.

Cervical decidual reactions are microscopically differentiated from invasive nonkeratinizing squamous cell carcinoma by lack of significant nuclear atypia or mitotic figures, lack of association with CIN, and the absence of continuity with the surface epithelium. Decidual cells also have uniform bland nuclei, while the nuclei of nonkeratinizing squamous cell carcinoma exhibit coarsely clumped chromatin. It should be noted, however, that a malignant tumor and ectopic decidua may coexist in the same patient.

Placental site nodules are usually located immediately beneath the epithelial surface and appear as discrete, well-defined nodules with lobulated contours composed of intermediate trophoblasts. A few lesions are elongated parallel to the surface of the epithelium in a plaque-like configuration. The intermediate trophoblasts have an abundant and eosinophilic to amphophilic cytoplasm with poorly defined cytoplasmic borders (Figs. 30.3, 30.4). Most intermediate trophoblast cells are mononucleate, but occasionally binucleate or multinucleate forms were present. The trophoblastic nuclei are frequently large, irregular, and hyperchromatic. These cells, however, lack significant atypia and mitotic activity. A peripheral chronic inflammatory infiltrate rich in plasma cells is usually present. In addition, there is abundant eosinophilic extracellular material, which can be prominent as well as hyalinization, especially in the central portion of the lesion. This finding may be confused with a rare type of invasive squamous cell carcinoma of the cervix characterized by necrosis, hyalinization, and well-circumscribed margins. The presence of focal keratinization excludes the diagnosis of trophoblastic lesion. Although the placental site nodule may be found incidentally in a patient with squamous dysplasia or squamous cell carcinoma in situ, there is no continuity between the two processes as there commonly is between dysplasia/carcinoma in situ and invasive squamous cell carcinoma. The lack of significant atypia and the presence of only rare mitotic figures favors placental site nodule over squamous cell carcinoma (Figs. 30.5, 30.6).

IMMUNOHISTOCHEMISTRY

In difficult cases, immunohistochemistry against keratin protein can be used to differentiate keratin-negative decidual reaction from keratin-positive squamous cell carcinoma. Intermediate trophoblasts, however, react strongly with antibodies against keratin, and a positive immunostain does not assist in the differential diagnosis between placental site nodule and squamous cell carcinoma. Intermediate trophoblasts also stain strongly and diffusely for placental alkaline phosphatase (PLAP), which is only rarely observed in carcinoma.

PROGNOSIS AND TREATMENT

Regression of cervical decidual reaction is observed after pregnancy, and the lesion usually disappears by 2 months postpartum.

Placental site nodules are important only in that if the lesion is not recognized, or differentiation from a more aggressive lesion such as placental site trophoblastic tumor is not achieved, a hysterectomy may be performed for these lesions.

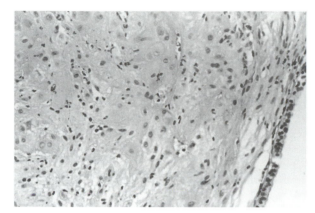

Figure 30.1. Decidual reaction of cervical stroma.

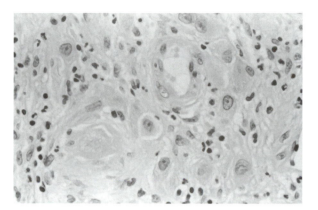

Figure 30.2. Decidmalized cervical stromal cells.

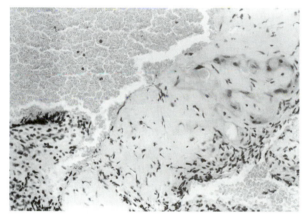

Figure 30.3. Placental site nodule detected in an ECC specimen.

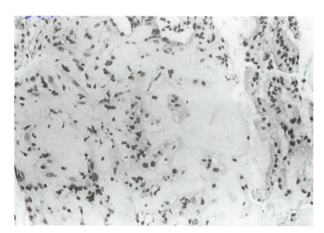

Figure 30.4. Placental site nodule.

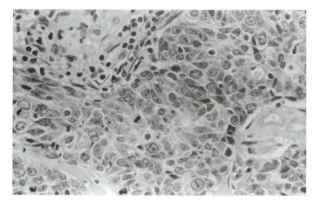

Figure 30.5. Squamous cell carcinoma.

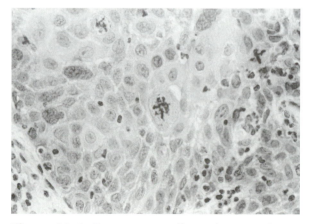

Figure 30.6. Squamous cell carcinoma. Contrast the cytologic features with those of decidualized cells and placental site nodule.

31. Small Cell (Neuroendocrine) Carcinoma

vs.

Squamous Cell Carcinoma of the Small Cell Nonkeratinizing Type

CLINICAL

Small cell undifferentiated carcinoma accounts for 2–5% of all cervical tumors. The median age of patients varies in different studies from 36 to 42 years, a decade younger than patients with nonkeratinizing squamous cell carcinoma. The presenting symptoms are nonspecific and similar to those of other more common cervical cancers. Most patients present with abnormal vaginal bleeding, few patients with abdominal or back pain, and occasional patients are asymptomatic.

GROSS

In general, the gross examination of small cell undifferentiated carcinoma of the cervix is indistinguishable from other forms of squamous cell carcinoma. Many small cell carcinomas, however, are more often large, ulcerative, and more deeply infiltrative than small cell squamous cell carcinoma. A barrel-shaped cervix is often formed.

HISTOLOGY

Squamous cell carcinoma of the cervix has been traditionally divided into large cell keratinizing, large cell nonkeratinizing, and small cell carcinoma. These tumors are classified primarily on the basis of their appearance or routine light microscopy; however, because the majority, but not all, of the latter group exhibit neuroendocrine, not squamous, differentiation the term *small undifferentiated (neuroendocrine) carcinoma* has been generally preferred.

Small cell undifferentiated carcinoma is characterized by an extensive diffuse infiltration of the cervical stroma by extremely cellular, closely packed small cells. These cells are arranged in poorly defined small nests, sheets, and trabeculae (Fig. 31.1). They have scant cytoplasm and oval–round to spindle nuclei. Nuclear molding may be prominent. The nuclei are hyperchromatic with evenly dispersed chromatinic material and inconspicu-

ous nucleoli. Intermediate cells with slightly large cytoplasm and irregular nuclei with occasional nucleoli may be observed. Nuclear detail in small cell undifferentiated carcinomas may be frequently obscured by extensive smudging or crush artifact (Figs. 31.2 and 31.3). Mitotic figures are usually numerous. Focal or broad zones of necrosis may be present. In addition, characteristic deposition of hematoxylin (Azzopardi phenomenon) around vessels may be observed. A minor component of squamous cell carcinoma or adenocarcinoma may be observed; however, this should not constitute more than 5–10% of the tumor volume. Tumors with more than 10% squamous glandular differentiation may be regarded as having mixed components.

The cells of squamous cell nonkeratinizing carcinoma with small cells have a high nucleus : cytoplasm ratio, but have more abundant cytoplasm and better-defined cellular borders than small cell undifferentiated carcinoma (Fig. 31.4). The nuclei are also larger and have coarse chromatin aggregates, which are separated by clear spaces. Nucleoli are readily visible. The cells generally resemble those of high-grade CIN and lack the nuclear molding and extensive crush artifact present in most small cell undifferentiated carcinomas (Figs. 31.5, 31.6). In addition, nonkeratinizing squamous carcinoma with small cells invades the stroma in discrete cohesive nests rather than diffusely in trabeculae or poorly defined nests as is characteristic for small cell undifferentiated carcinoma. Squamous cell carcinoma is usually associated with intense inflammatory and desmoplastic host response, which are usually lacking or minimal around small cell undifferentiated carcinoma.

ANCILLARY STUDIES

Ultrastructural studies can aid in the diagnosis of small cell undifferentiated carcinoma. Neuroendocrine dense-core granules, however, vary in quantity from one case to another and may require extensive search at the light-microscopy and ultrastructural levels. Positive immunohistochemistry for neuroendocrine markers such as chromogranin, neuron-specific enolase, and synaptophysin are present in most cases. Less commonly, a variety of polypeptides such as ACTH (adrenocorticotropic hormone), serotonin, calcitonin, gastrin, and somatostatin may be observed.

Ultrastructural studies and Immunohistochemistry, however, may not be as helpful because approximately 40% of nonkeratinizing squamous carcinoma with small cells are positive for neuroendocrine markers and an equal percentage of small cell undifferentiated carcinomas are positive for cytokeratins. Immunohistochemical staining for the monoclonal antibody, referred to as *squamous cell carcinoma antigen* or "PA-4," is linked to squamous differentiation and keratinization and may assist in this differential diagnosis.

PROGNOSIS AND TREATMENT

Small cell undifferentiated carcinomas (small and intermediate cell types) are highly aggressive neoplasms associated with poor prognosis. They have the propensity to metastasize early and widely by both lymphatic and hematogenous routes. The prognosis of the tumor is worse than that of stage-comparable nonkeratinizing squamous cell carcinoma with small cells. Clinical stage does not correlate as well with survival as it does in patients with squamous cell carcinoma indicating high frequency of occult metastasis at the time of presentation. The currently recommended therapy includes combinations of radiation and chemotherapy with or without radical hysterectomy.

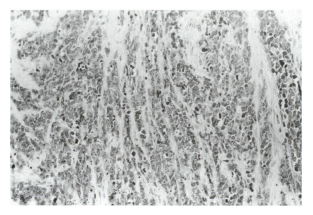

Figure 31.1. Small cell undifferentiated carcinoma.

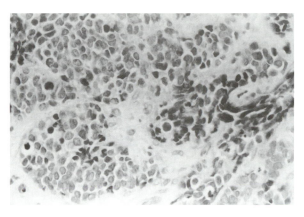

Figure 31.2. Small cell undiffeentiated carcinoma. Note nuclear molding and crush artifact.

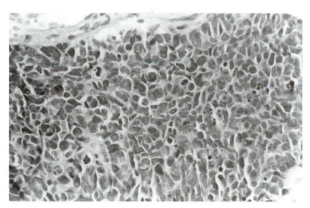

Figure 31.3. Small cell undifferentiated carcinoma.

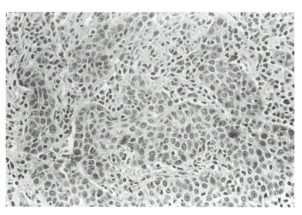

Figure 31.4. Squamous cell non-keratinizing carcinoma with small cells.

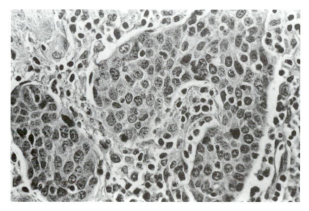

Figure 31.5. Squamous cell non-keratinizing carcinoma with small cells.

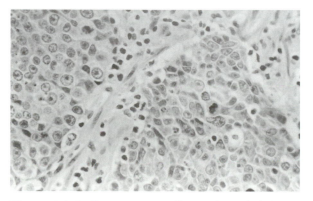

Figure 31.6. Squamous cell non-keratinizing carcinoma with small cells.

32. Endometriosis of Endocervix
vs.
Tubule Metaplasia
vs.
Endocervical Carcinoma in situ

CLINICAL

Superficial endometriosis of the cervix typically develops in adult women between the ages of 20 and 50 years. The condition may be an asymptomatic incidental finding or associated with postcoital bleeding, premenstrual spotting, and less commonly, menorrhagia. Almost all patients have had prior cervical trauma such as cone biopsy, electrocautery, and dilatation and curettage of the endometrium. This association has led most investigators to favor implantation as the most significant pathogenic mechanism. In contrast, deep or secondary cervical endometriosis is usually a continuous extension of endometriosis of the rectovaginal septum, serosa of the supravaginal portion of the cervix, or involvement of the cul de sac in association with more widespread pelvic endometriosis. These patients present with palpable cysts or nodules deep in the posterior wall of the cervix.

Tubal metaplasia of the endocervix is usually encountered as an incidental finding on cervical cytology, biopsies, and hysterectomies performed on women in the reproductive age group for a variety of clinical situations, including CIN or abnormal uterine bleeding. It has been estimated to occur in approximately 30% of hysterectomy specimens but is probably more commonly present in cases in which many tissue blocks are submitted for microscopic examination.

The mean age of women with adrenocarcinoma in situ (AIS) of the endocervix is 36 to 39 years; a decade or two younger than those with invasive adenocarcinoma. Most women with AIS are asymptomatic, and the lesion is detected either during cytologic screening or unexpectedly on an endocervical curettage, cervical punch biopsy, or cone/LEEP biopsy performed during the workup for CIN or in hysterectomy specimens removed for a variety of unrelated conditions. In women who are symptomatic, the symptoms, such as abnormal vaginal bleeding or discharge, are usually related to other gynecologic conditions.

GROSS

Superficial endometriosis presents as solitary or multiple friable, dark red or brown patches, nodules, or cysts measuring a few millimeters in diameter. Prior to menses, these lesions may enlarge and become blue or purple. During menses, they may rupture resulting in an irregular ulcer. Rarely, these lesions become puckered secondary to fibrosis.

Endocervical tubal metaplasia is typically found high in the cervical canal and does not present with any recognizable gross features.

AIS has no distinctive gross features. It often lies superior to the squamocolumnar junction, outside the transformation zone, and is seldom visible colposcopically. When visible, the epithelium may be only slightly thicker, with the crypts more irregular than normal.

HISTOLOGY

Superficial endometriosis of the cervix is characterized by the presence of endometrial glands surrounded by endometrial stroma (Fig. 32.1). The lesions are usually located in the superficial lamina propria and should have no connection with the adjacent endometrium. Stromal endometriosis is an uncommon lesion characterized by the presence of well-circumscribed foci within the superficial stroma of the cervix that are exclusively composed of closely packed cells resembling endometrial stromal cells, small blood vessels, and extravasated erythrocytes (Fig. 32.2).

Tubal metaplasia is characterized by the replacement of the endocervical surface epithelium and/or clefts by a müllerian-type epithelium that closely resembles that of the fallopian tube and often contains all three cell types (ciliated, secretory, and intercalated) (Fig. 32.3). The architecture of the clefts showing tubal metaplasia is similar to that of normal endocervical clefts. Ciliated cells are the predominant cell type in tubal metaplasia. The secretory cells have a high nucleus : cytoplasm ratio and their nuclei tend to be oval to round and slightly larger and more hyperchromatic than those of the normal endocervical cells (Fig. 32.4). Nonsecretory cells with cilia are normally found in the lining epithelium of the endocervix, especially high in the endocervical canal; however, this does not represent tubal metaplasia because of the absence of the various cell types present in the normal fallopian tube.

AIS is characterized by partial or complete replacement of the surface glandular epithelium and/or endocervical crypts by cytologically abnormal epithelial cells (Fig. 32.5). The crypts are normally situated in the cervix and are or normal size and shape, but they reveal cellular stratification, loss of polarity, and loss of cytoplasmic mucin. AIS lesions demonstrate striking nuclear crowding, enlargement, hyperchromasia, and prominent mitotic activity. The degree of stratification in AIS may be so prominent as to produce discrete papillary projections, intraluminal bridges, and a cribform pattern (Fig. 32.6). Typically, there is a sharp demarcation of AIS from uninvolved glands and from the uninvolved epithelium of the same glands.

Endocervical, intestinal, and endometrioid types of AIS have been reported; the vast majority of cases are of the endocervical type. Intestinal AIS is characterized by the presence of goblet cells; however, argyrophilic cells may also be present. Endometrioid AIS is characterized by cells with scanty cytoplasm, marked nuclear pseudostratification, and absent intracytoplasmic mucin.

Superficial endometriosis may mimic AIS; however, the former is characterized by glands lined by endometrial-like cells with basally oriented nuclei that do not demonstrate nuclear atypia. These glands are surrounded by endometrial-type stroma, which, although occasionally may be scant, establishes the diagnosis of endometriosis.

Tubal metaplasia can also be confused with AIS because of the presence of pseudostratification, mild cytologic atypia, and high nucleus : cytoplasm ratio. The lack of true nuclear stratification, dispolarity, nuclear atypia, and mitotic activity helps differentiate tubule metaplasia from AIS. Most importantly, the presence of ciliated cells in tubal metaplasia serves to differentiate it from AIS.

PROGNOSIS AND TREATMENT

Cervical endometriosis may be managed by excision or electrocautarization.

Tubal metaplasia does not require specific treatment; however, it is important to recognize it and distinguish it from other lesions that it mimics and that do require specific therapy.

Several investigators have used or proposed conization as acceptable conservative therapy for AIS. The optimum conization method to excise AIS for diagnosis and treatment should encompass all the transformation zone and should have clear margins. If retention of reproductive potential is not desired, then a simple hysterectomy may be performed.

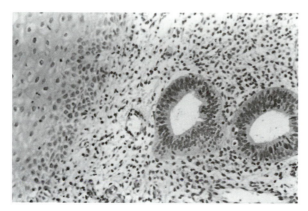

Figure 32.1. Cervical endometriosis.

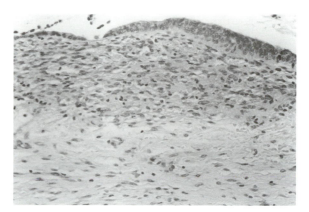

Figure 32.2. Stromal endometriosis.

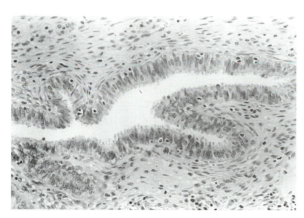

Figure 32.3. Tubal metaplasia.

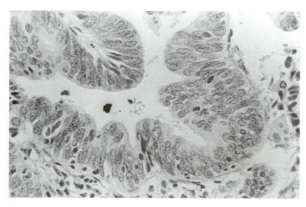

Figure 32.4. Tubule metaplasia.

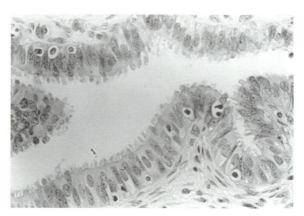

Figure 32.5. Adenocarcinoma in situ of endocervical epithelium.

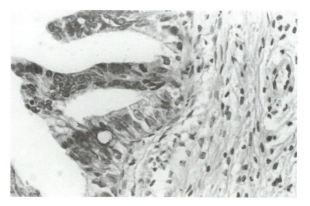

Figure 32.6. Adenocarcinoma in situ of endocervical epithelium.

33. Adenocarcinoma in situ of Endocervix

vs.

Early Invasive Adenocarcinoma of Endocervix

CLINICAL

Retrospective studies of cervical smears and biopsies demonstrate that changes of adenocarcinoma in situ may precede invasive adenocarcinoma in 10–25% of cases. The mean age for a woman with endocervical adenocarcinoma in situ has been reported to range from 36 to 39 years old, compared to 48–53 years for those with invasive adenocarcinoma. Patients with early invasive carcinoma have been reported to have a mean age of 40–44 years and are usually asymptomatic.

GROSS

Most of the adenocarcinomas in situ and early invasive adenocarcinoma are not visible clinically or colposcopically and are detected by an abnormal cervical smears or random cervical biopsies. About 50–60% of in situ invasive adenocarcinoma have coexisting CIN on cervical smears. These cell changes may obscure those of adenocarcinoma.

HISTOLOGY

Because of problems in defining criteria as well as histologic difficulties, the existence of early (microinvasive) adenocarcinoma as an entity remains in dispute. Some investigators define early adenocarcinoma as that involving cervical stroma to a depth of <5 mm as measured from the mucosal surface of the endocervical canal and others have used volume measurements (<500 mm^3). Measurement of a lateral extent (≤7 mm) with separation of early invasive lesions into those showing minimal stromal invasions (<1 mm) and microinvasive carcinomas has also been employed. Still others do not recognize microinvasive adenocarcinoma as an entity, and any infiltrative lesion is considered a full-fledged invasive adenocarcinoma irrespective of the depth of invasion.

Important histopathologic clues to the presence of invasion include the following (Figs. 33.1–33.6):

1. Abnormal glandular architectural pattern, specifically, the presence of infiltrating glands that lack the normal lobular architecture of endocervical glands with AIS.
2. Extension of neoplastic glands significantly deeper than that of adjacent normal endocervical glands or beyond the usual confines of normal endocervical glands.
3. The presence of poorly formed small neoplastic glands with irregular configurations and/or orientations that are different from that expected in normal endocervix or in the cervix involved by AIS (Fig. 33.2, 33.4).
4. The glands may be arranged in a monotonous group or parallel rows that are juxtaposed or confluent in a complex back-to-back pattern without intervening stroma. Tongue-like processes at the periphery of glands involved by AIS are present (Fig. 33.6). This budding and branching of affected glands is characteristic of early invasion.
5. Small nests of cells in the stroma or small buds of squamoid cells with eosinophilic cytoplasm projecting into the stroma. These small buds of squamoid cells contain abundant eosinophilic cytoplasm and enlarged round nuclei with chromatin clearing and prominent nucleoli. With progression, these buds form microacini.

Invasion usually elicits an inflammatory or desmoplastic response; however, this may be absent. The histologic assessment of early stromal invasion, however, remains difficult and occasionally subjective, and in some cases it may not be impossible to distinguish AIS from early invasive carcinoma.

PROGNOSIS AND TREATMENT

The natural history of AIS and invasive adenocarcinoma is poorly understood. It appears that many patients with AIS can be managed by cone biopsy alone, but it is important for the pathologist to carefully assess and report adequacy of the cone biopsy margins. Some, however, regard hysterectomy as the preferred treatment option, as cone biopsy appears to carry significant risk of residual disease. Until extensive data to the contrary are available, measurable small invasive adenocarcinoma is usually treated more aggressively.

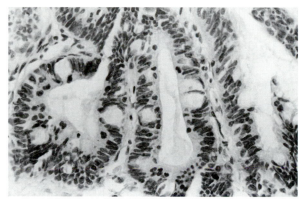

Figure 33.1. Adenocarcinoma in situ of endocervical epithelium, intestinal type.

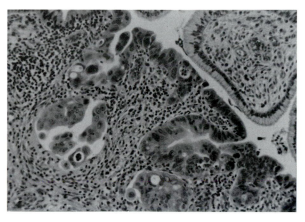

Figure 33.2. Early invasive adenocarcinoma of endocervix.

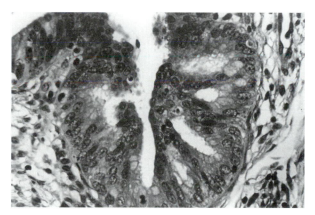

Figure 33.3. Adenocarcinoma in situ of endocervical epithelium.

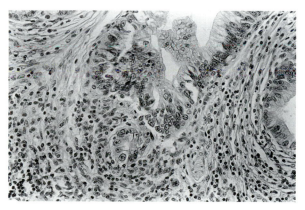

Figure 33.4. Adenocarcinoma in situ of endocervical epithelium with early invasive component. Inflammatory and fibrous response.

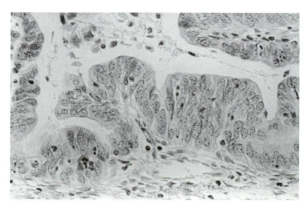

Figure 33.5. Adenocarcinoma in situ of endocervical epithelium.

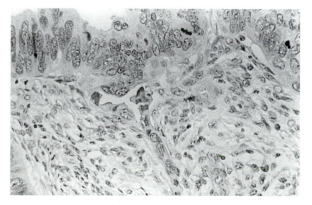

Figure 33.6. Early invasive adenocarcinoma of endocervix.

34. Low-Grade Endocervical Glandular Dysplasia/Atypia

vs.

High-Grade Endocervical Dysplasia/Atypia

CLINICAL

As with squamous carcinoma in situ, it may be expected that adenocarcinoma in situ is preceded by precursor lesions of lesser severity. These precursor lesions described as endocervical glandular dysplasia or atypia represent a spectrum of changes, with adenocarcinoma in situ representing the most severe lesion in this spectrum. In addition, the finding that the mean age of patients with cervical glandular dysplasia was less than that generally reported for patients with AIS suggests that there is a progression through increasing degrees of glandular dysplasia to adenocarcinoma in situ. Endocervical glandular dysplasia, however, is rarely detected as an isolated finding, and its natural history remains to be further elucidated. Sharp division between these two lesions is not possible as diagnostic criteria are subjective and have been poorly defined.

HISTOLOGY

Endocervical glandular dysplasia defines a lesion in which the glands in an uninflamed region of the cervix are architecturally unremarkable but display moderate nuclear enlargement, hyperchromasia, and atypia (Figs. 34.1-34.6). The nuclear stratification, mitotic activity, and cytologic atypia are less than those of AIS. These glands are usually lined by two to three layers of cells. The nuclei are enlarged round to oval and retain polarity. They show mild to moderate irregularity and hyperchromasia. The nuclear stratification, mitotic activity, and cytologic atypia are less than those of adenocarcinoma in situ. Cribriform glands and papillary formations, characteristic of AIS, are usually absent in endocervical dysplasia (Figs. 34.4, 34.5). The cells are not clearly cytologically malignant.

In addition, the changes of endocervical dysplasia are focal. If the cells are markedly atypical but only one gland is involved, a diagnosis of endocervical dysplasia is favored over AIS (Fig. 34.5). Adenocarcinoma in situ usually involves the endocervical surface epithelium and the glandular clefts, and often is multifocal in several histologic sections (Fig. 34.6).

Some investigators have suggested that the glandular lesions with less atypia than in AIS could be grouped into low- or high-grade dysplasias; the latter group often were found to border adenocarcinoma in situ. The distinction between high-grade dysplasia and AIS, however, may be arbitrary. Others advocate placing all lesions regarded as less than AIS in a glandular dysplasia category without division into subcategories.

There is only limited experience with the management of glandular dysplasia. In itself, it does not appear to be an indication for hysterectomy. Conservative management approach with follow-up is preferred.

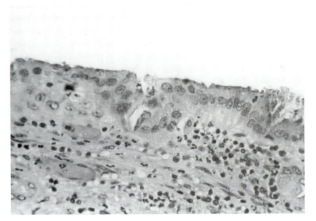

Figure 34.1. Inflammatory type atypia of endocervical epithelium.

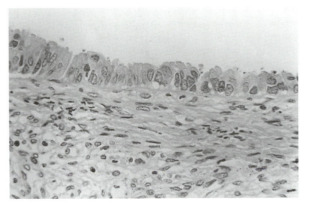

Figure 34.2. Endocervical glandular dysplasia of surface epithelium.

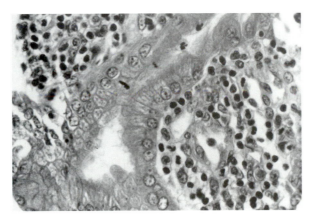

Figure 34.3. Reative/inflammatory changes bordering on endocervical glandular dysplasia, low grade.

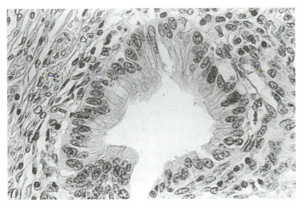

Figure 34.4. Endocervical glandular dysplasia.

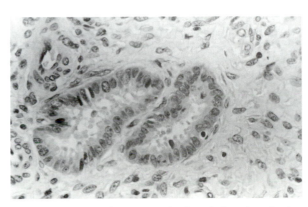

Figure 34.5. Endocervical glandular dysplasia. Single focus observed in a cervical core biopsy.

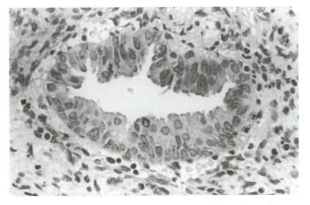

Figure 34.6. Endocervical glandular dysplasia; high graade/adenocarcinoma in situ.

35. Deep Nabothian Cysts
vs.
Tunnel Clusters
vs.
Minimal Deviation Adenocarcinoma (Adenoma Malignum)

CLINICAL

Nabothian cysts of the cervix develop within the transformation zone secondary to squamous metaplasia covering over and obstructing the cervical clefts. Deep Nabothian cysts are usually incidental findings in patients who undergo cone biopsies or hysterectomy for a variety of disease processes.

Tunnel clusters are benign collections of endocervical glands that usually are located close to the surface of the epithelium of the cervix. The lesions are uncommon before the age of 30. They have been reported in the transformation zone in 8% of all adult women, 13% postmenopausal women, and 40% of women in the first trimester of pregnancy. When endocervical tunnel clusters are prominent, the patient almost always proves to be multigravida. The patients are asymptomatic, and the lesion is usually detected as an incidental finding in either cone biopsies or hysterectomy specimens performed for unrelated reasons.

Minimal deviation adenocarcinomas or adenoma malignum account for only 1–3% of all cervical adenocarcinoma. They occur in patients ranging in age from 25 to 72 years with an average of 42 years. The most common presenting symptom is menometrorrhagia followed by mucoid or watery vaginal discharge. In a number of patients the cervical tumor may occur synchronously or prior to the development of ovarian tumors, which are usually mucinous neoplasms or the rare ovarian sex cord tumors with annular tubules. Both minimal deviation adenocarcinoma of the cervix and ovarian sex cord tumors with annular tubules have also been strongly associated with the Peutz–Jeghers (after J.L.A. Peutz and H.Jeghers) syndrome.

GROSS

Grossly deep Nabothian cysts appear as yellow or white mucin-filled cysts that are frequently multiple and may measure ≤1.0 cm in diameter. Large cysts may result in gross enlargement of the cervix.

Endocervical tunnel clusters usually result in distortion of the endocervix by mucin-filled retention cysts of various sizes. These cysts are usually multifocal and may extend deep into the wall of the cervix. They range in size from 0.5 to 2.0 cm in diameter. In some patients no gross lesions are observed.

The cervix in minimal deviation adenocarcinoma is typically firm and indurated. The mucosal surface may be hemorrhagic, friable, or mucoid. The carcinomas may be ulcerated or polypoid but often form a suspicious-appearing irregularity, or the cervix may be stenotic without any obvious lesion. With early lesions, the cervix can appear normal.

HISTOLOGY

Nabothian cysts are generally located immediately beneath the endocervix or metaplastic epithelium, but occasionally they can lie as deep as 8 or 9 mm in the cervical stroma and be designated as deep Nabothian cysts (Fig. 35.1). These deep cysts may extend through the endocervix to within 1 mm of the paracervical connective tissue. However, they do not have an irregular infiltrative pattern and do not vary markedly in size and shape. The cysts are lined by a single layer of endocervical-type cells that vary from columnar to flattened (Fig. 35.2). The lining epithelium is almost always at least focally positive for mucicarmine stain. Squamous metaplasia of the lining epithelium may occur. Mitotic figures, cell stratification, or a stromal reaction are not observed. Deep Nabothian glands do not incite a desmplastic stromal response.

Tunnel clusters are characterized by the presence of an organized, lobular, or nodular aggregate of closely packed, uniform, round, tubular, or cystically dilated endocervical glands (Fig. 35.3). Endocervical tunnel clusters have well-demarcated borders, are oval or rounded in shape, and do not extend beyond the depth of normal endocervical glands. Connections between the "tunnels" and endocervical clefts and Nabothian cysts are often present.

The tunnels are lined by a single layer of flat, cuboidal, or low-columnar epithelial endocervical-type cells (Fig. 35.4). Their lumina may contain inspissated mucous fluid. Small foci of extravasated mucin from ruptured tunnels are frequently seen. Some glands demonstrate orderly branching and short, slender papillary enfoldings. There is no epithelial stratification, atypia, or loss of polarity. Intraglandular bridges, cribriform patterns, mitotic figures, or an invasive pattern are absent. Inflammatory and reparative changes, however, may be observed.

Minimal deviation adenocarcinoma is characterized by the presence of cytologically low-grade or bland glands with an abnormal architectural appearance that exhibit deep invasion of the cervical wall (Fig. 35.5). The glands vary in size and shape from small and round to large, irregular, and distorted forms with complex convolutions. Occasionally, the glands are cystically dilated and may exhibit papillary epithelial enfoldings. The deeper glands are not oriented toward the surface and infiltrate the stroma in a haphazard fashion. Most of the glands are lined by a single layer of mucin-containing columnar epithelial cells with bland basal nuclei that show minimal, if any, nuclear atypia (Fig. 35.6). Some tumors may display an endometrioid or clear cell differentiation. Most neoplasms show at least occasional glands that are lined by obviously malignant epithelia that show nuclear atypia with enlargement, chromatin clumping, and occasional nucleoli. Increased mitotic activity may be observed in these areas of less well-differentiated adenocarcinoma. Minimal deviation adenocarcinoma may underlie normal squamous or endocervical epithelium, but the surface epithelium may show hyperplastic appearance of glands similar to villous adenoma of the colon. A desmoplastic stromal response is usually present around at least some of the angulated glands and may be a prominent feature. Mucin pools with granulation tissue response and mucin-containing macrophages may be observed. Encroachment of blood vessels and nerve fibers by invasive glands may be present in a significant number of cases. The diagnosis of minimal deviation adenocarcinoma can be extremely difficult because deep positioning of the glands is needed to confirm invasion. Often, the diagnosis requires a deep cone or hysterectomy.

Adenoma malignum should also be distinguished from benign endocervical adenomyomas. The latter are grossly well circumscribed and polypoid with lobular arrangement of endocervical-type glands, admixed with smooth muscle. Endocervical adenomyomas lack glandular invasion, desmoplastic reaction, or cytologic atypia and are benign lesions.

PROGNOSIS AND TREATMENT

Deep Nabothian cysts are nonneoplastic lesions, and their sole significance is in that they may mimic histopathologically an adenocarcinoma.

Tunnel clusters do not represent a hyperplastic or premalignant change and probably represent an evolutional stage of the normal endocervical clefts/glands. They have no clinical significance.

The majority of reports of minimal deviation adenocarcinoma document an unfavorable survival rate, but most neoplasms are discovered in late stages. Many fail to form visibly evident lesions despite deep infiltration leading to great opportunity for vascular invasion and clinical understaging, resulting in undertreatment and a relatively poor prognosis. Some studies, however, report the survival rate to be similar to that for other forms of well-differentiated adenocarcinoma of the cervix at the same stage. The distribution of metastasis is similar to that of other cervical adenocarcinomas.

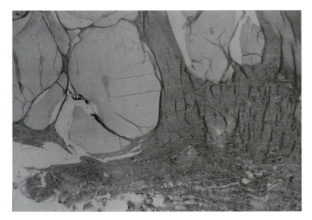

Figure 35.1. Deep nobothian cysts.

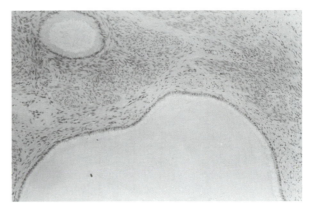

Figure 35.2. Deep nobothian cysts.

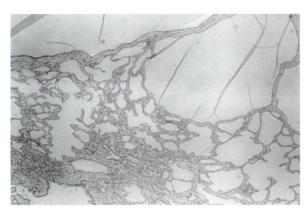

Figure 35.3. Tunnel clusters.

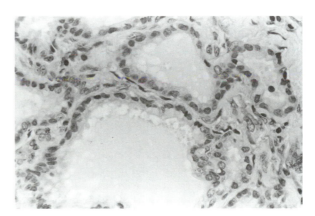

Figure 35.4. Tunnel clusters.

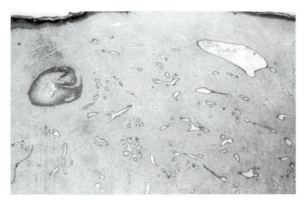

Figure 35.5. Minimal deviation adenocarcinoma (adenoma malignum).

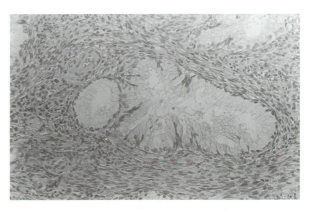

Figure 35.6. Minimal deviation adenocarcinoma (adenoma malignum).

36. Well-Differentiated Villoglandular Adenocarcinoma

vs.

Primary Endocervical Papillary Serous Carcinoma

CLINICAL

Most patients with well-differentiated villoglandular adenocarcinoma are <40 years of age, with the average age range from different studies, of 33–37 years. This contrasts with an average age in the late 40s and early 50s for patients with the other more common types of cervical adenocarcinomas. Villoglandular adenocarcinoma has frequently been associated with the use of oral contraceptives. The patients may present with abnormal vaginal bleeding; however, some are asymptomatic and investigated because of an abnormal cytologic smear.

Only a few documented cases of primary papillary serous adenocarcinoma of the uterine cervix have been reported. The rarity of this lesion does not yet allow for specification of the age distribution or presenting symptoms. The presentation, however, appears to be similar to other types of adenocarcinoma in that most patients present with abnormal bleeding and a few are asymptomatic and investigated for the presence of an abnormal cytology smear.

GROSS

Well-differentiated villoglandular adenocarcinoma usually appears as a polypoid or broad-based papillary protuberance ranging in diameter from 0.5 to 3.5 cm and may resemble a polyp or condyloma accuminatum. Some tumors are more subtle, however, presenting as an eroded or friable cervical enlargement.

The few reports of primary endocervical papillary serous carcinoma have documented the presence of a friable hemorrhagic tumor in the endocervix.

HISTOLOGY

Well-differentiated villoglandular carcinoma presents as a complex branching or arborescent pattern of orderly villous-like papillary fronds (Fig. 36.1). The fronds are usually long and thin but may be of variable size or thick and short. These branching papillae give rise to smaller branching processes. They contain a central core of fibromatosis stroma composed of spindle-shaped cells resembling endocervical stroma. The fibrous cords may contain

variable numbers of acute and chronic inflammatory cells. The papillary processes are lined by a low-stratified epithelial cells that may be endocervical, endometrioid, or intestinal type (Fig. 36.2). The latter may include goblet cells. Typically, there is slight to moderate nuclear atypia (Fig. 36.3). The lesions are usually well circumscribed, and the invasive portions are a continuation of the elongated branching glands. They are separated by a minimal stromal response, which may be desmoplastic or myxoid, that involves the advancing margin of the islands. The term *well-differentiated villoglandular adenocarcinoma* should be reserved for tumors in which the villoglandular pattern is the exclusive or almost the exclusive one. Unlike other types of papillary adenocarcinoma, well-differentiated villoglandular adenocarcinoma is characterized by a less complex, more orderly papillae and by minimal epithelial budding. Cellular stratification is mild, psammoma bodies are absent and the nuclear features are low-grade, features that are in sharp contrast to those of papillary serous adenocarcinoma.

The histologic features of primary endocervical papillary serous carcinoma are identical to those of papillary serous adenocarcinomas arising in the ovary or endometrium (Fig. 36.4). The tumors are composed of papillary tufts and complex papillae with central fibrovascular cores. Numerous fine cellular and irregular papillae and detached cellular buds are evident. The papillae are lined by atypical markedly stratified cuboidal epithelial cells with moderate amounts of eosinophilic cytoplasm. The tumor cells have pleomorphic high-grade nuclear features. (Figs. 36.5, 36.6). Occasional nuclei have prominent nucleoli. Mitotic figures are usually numerous. Minor foci of necrosis may be present. Other less prominent features include irregular slit-like glandular spaces and solid nests or sheets of cells in the deeper invasive component of the tumor. A minor component of the tumor may be similar to well-differentiated villoglandular papillary adenocarcinoma.

PROGNOSIS AND TREATMENT

The majority of well-differentiated villoglandular adenocarcinomas are superficially invasive; however, deep invasion with extension into the uterine corpus may occur. A therapeutic cervical cone has been suggested in young patients desirous of maintaining fertility and in whom the invasion is <3 mm and there is no vascular space invasion or involvement of resection margins. In general, the clinical outcome of patients with well-differentiated villoglandular adenocarcinoma has been excellent. Radical surgery and adjuvant therapy do not appear to be necessary for treatment of the great majority of these cases.

It is not possible to draw definite conclusions regarding the behavior of endocervical papillary serous carcinoma from the study of only a few cases. There is evidence, however, to suggest that although these lesions may not be deeply invasive, they are more aggressive than endocervical adenocarcinoma of the usual types. Few patients presented with nodal metastasis despite superficial invasion. This tendency for more aggressive behavior may be similar to that of papillary serous adenocarcinoma of the endometrium. The diagnosis of papillary serous carcinoma of the cervix should be made only after spread from the ovaries, fallopian tubes, and endometrium has been excluded.

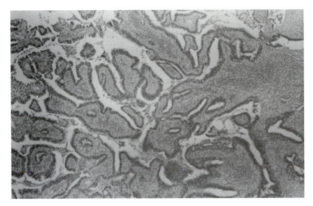

Figure 36.1. Well-differentiated Villoglandular adenocarcinoma.

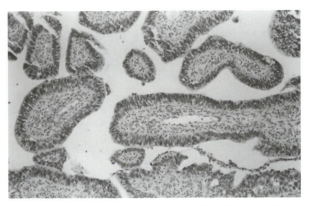

Figure 36.2. Well-differentiated Villoglandular adenocarcinoma.

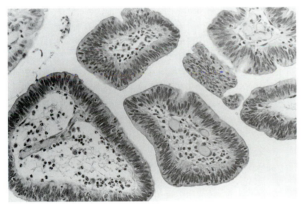

Figure 36.3. Well-differentiated Villoglandular adenocarcinoma.

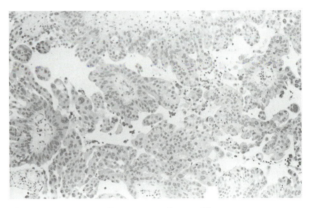

Figure 36.4. Endocervical papillary serous adenocarcinoma.

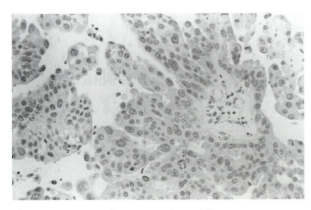

Figure 36.5. Endocervical papillary serous adenocarcinoma.

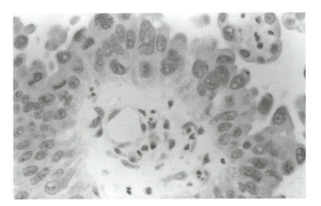

Figure 36.6. Endocervical papillary serous adenocarcinoma.

37. Microglandular Hyperplasia

vs.

"Atypical," Microglandular Hyperplasia

vs.

Clear Cell Carcinoma

CLINICAL

Microglandular hyperplasia is most common in women in the reproductive age group, with a mean age of 33.5 years. It is usually related to progesterone stimulation, most commonly oral contraceptives and much less frequently during pregnancy. Approximately 6% of reported cases, however, have been in women who are neither on any hormonal preparation nor pregnant. It has even been reported in postmenopausal women, some of whom have been exposed to estrogen–progesterone therapy and others who have had coexisting endometrial hyperplasia or carcinoma. Patients with microglandular hyperplasia are usually asymptomatic but may complain of abnormal vaginal bleeding, spotting, or vaginal discharge.

Approximately half of clear cell carcinoma of the cervix can be linked to a history of maternal DES exposure and occur in young women, usually in their teens. The tumor may develop in the absence of DES exposure at any age, but particularly in older postmenopausal women. The clinical presentation is similar to that of other types of cervical carcinoma, and vaginal bleeding is the most common complaint.

GROSS

Microglandular hyperplasia is usually an incidental finding encountered in up to 27% of cervical cone biopsies or hysterectomy specimens. Its frequency may be higher in patients with a history of oral contraceptive use. Large lesions, however, may be grossly visible as an erosion, polypoid, or nodular friable lesion that may be single or multiple. These lesions may simulate an endocervical polyp. Early lesions may appear sessile.

The majority of clear cell adenocarcinomas present as nodular or polypoid fungating reddish lesions. Occasionally, there may be little abnormality of overlying mucosa or small punctate ulcers. Sporadically developing tumors arise in either the ecto- or endocervix, whereas tumors developing in DES exposed women invariably develop on the ectocervix.

HISTOLOGY

The surface and/or deeper portions of the endocervical cleft in microglandular hyperplasia is replaced focally or in multiple areas by densely crowded proliferation of glands that vary in size from small and round to irregularly dilated cystic structures (Fig. 37.1). This complex proliferation of glands is occasionally separated by scanty to abundant fibrous stroma, which is rarely extensively hyalinized. The glands and cysts are usually lined by a single layer of low-columnar, cuboidal, or flat epithelial cells that contain varying amounts of mucin. The cells have small to moderate amounts of clear, pale, to finely granular basophilic cytoplasm and typically show subnuclear vacuoles that may stain for mucin and may be conspicuous (Fig. 37.2). The nuclei are almost always uniform, small, and round to oval, with an evenly disbursed chromatin pattern. These nuclei occasionally protrude into the lumen of the gland and cysts in a hobnail pattern. Nucleoli are occasionally present. Mitotic figures are generally absent or sparse. Nuclear enlargement, hyperchromasia, and slight irregularity may be present, especially in pregnancy or as a degenerative change. The glands and cysts may show small foci of reserve cell hyperplasia and squamous metaplasia that occasionally may be prominent, resulting in a complex pattern. Their luminae usually contain a basophilic or eosinophilic secretion that stain for mucin. Neutrophils are typically present in the glands and can be very conspicuous in the intervening stroma. Less often, chronic inflammatory cells and occasionally eosinophils may be observed in the stroma.

Occasionally "atypical forms" of microglandular hyperplasia pose difficult diagnostic problems (Figs. 37.3, 37.4). The clinical presentation of these lesions is similar to that of conventional microglandular hyperplasia; however, they are more likely to be larger and present as polypoid cervical lesions in symptomatic women. These atypical patterns represent extremes in the spectrum of this benign condition and have been described as solid, mucinous, reticular, or hyalinized. The solid pattern is characterized by solid sheets, nests, and chords of cells with slight vacuolated cytoplasm. The cells have more abundant eosinophilic cytoplasm than that of typical foci of microglandular hyperplasia. The nuclei may be centrally positioned or slightly eccentric, giving a similarity to signet-ring carcinoma. The mucinous pattern shows occasional scattered cells, islands and nests of cells that have abundant mucinous cytoplasm and appear to float in the pools of mucin. The reticular pattern is characterized by the presence of cells, some of which are spindle-shaped, which are loosely dispersed in an edematous stromal background. The hyalinized pattern shows abundant stromal hyalinization. In general, however, although there may be slight nuclear atypia, the nuclear features in the "atypical patterns" are bland and are usually similar to those of the typical microglandular hyperplasia. Mitoses are also absent or extremely rare. Stromal invasion is absent. It is important to note that these unusual patterns are generally associated or merge with typical areas of microglandular hyperplasia, facilitating their recognition.

Microglandular hyperplasia should be diagnosed with caution in a postmenopausal patient, particularly if the findings are present in endometrial curettings. These cases may represent uterine adenocarcinomas that has been reported to simulate microglandular hyperplasia histologically.

The histologic features of clear cell adenocarcinoma in young patients with known exposure to DES are similar to those noted in older women without DES exposure. Clear cell adenocarcinoma has three basic patterns:

tubulocystic, solid, and papillary (Fig. 37.5). Although a mixture of several patterns is not uncommon, in a given tumor one particular pattern usually predominates. The predominant cells have abundant, clear, or eosinophilic granular cytoplasm. The clearing is the result of accumulation of abundant glycogen. The cells often have a hobnail shape in that they have scant cytoplasm and prominent hyperchromatic and pleomorphic nuclei that project into the lumen of the cysts and tubules (Fig. 37.6). Mitotic figures are easily recognized. Most clear cell carcinomas of the cervix are usually closely associated with vaginal adenosis or cervical ectropion.

TREATMENT AND PROGNOSIS

Microglandular hyperplasia is usually a benign incidental finding. Most importantly, the pathologist should be aware of its spectrum of manifestation to avoid misinterpretation as a malignant tumor. No patients have been reported to develop malignant tumors on long-term follow up.

Most patients with clear cell carcinoma are at stage I or II when detected. Treatment is either radical hysterectomy and vaginectomy or radiation. Features associated with a better prognosis include older age of patients, small size of the tumor, shallow depth of invasion, and a tubulocystic microscopic pattern. The prognosis is relatively good, and the survival rate is approximately 55% and 40% at 5 and 10 years, respectively.

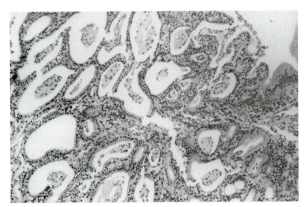

Figure 37.1. Microglandular hyperplasia of endocervix.

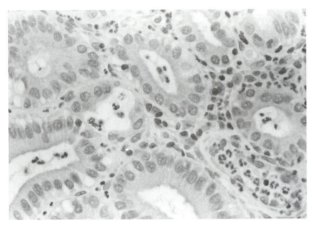

Figure 37.2. Microglandular hyperplasia of endocervix.

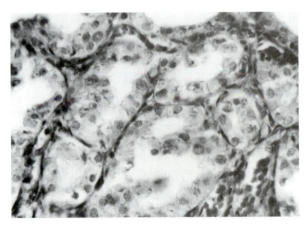

Figure 37.3. Microglandular hyperplasia with atypia.

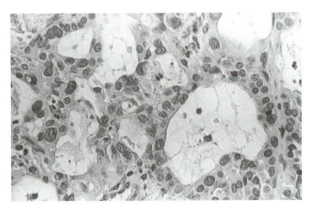

Figure 37.4. Microglandular hyperplasia with atypia.

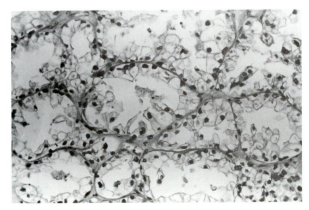

Figure 37.5. Clear cell adenocarcinoma.

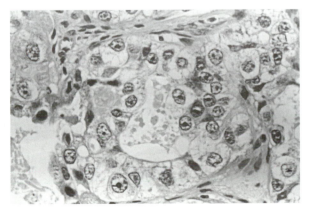

Figure 37.6. Clear cell adenocarcinoma.

38. Clear Cell Carcinoma

vs.

Cervical Arias-Stella Reaction

CLINICAL

Arias-Stella (after Javier Arias-Stella) reaction (ASR) occurs in the endometrium in association with intrauterine or extrauterine pregnancy and trophoblastic disease. Occasionally, however, it can occur in endocervical glands under the same circumstances. It has been reported in the endocervix in approximately 9% of gravid hysterectomy specimens. The clinical, gross, and histologic features of clear cell carcinoma are discussed in Chapter 37.

GROSS

ASR of endocervix does not manifest as a grossly detected lesion.

HISTOLOGY

The histopathologic features of Arias-Stella Reaction in the endocervical glands are identical to those that occur in the endometrium (Fig. 38.1). The reaction usually involves only a small number of glands but occasionally may be extensive. Involvement of superficial glands is more common than that of deep glands. Glands within an endocervical polyp may also be affected. The cells lining the glands may exhibit regular papillary processes or may be pseudostratified to the extent that they almost obliterate the lumen (Figs. 38.2, 38.3). The glands are lined by enlarged epithelial cells having hypersecretory cytoplasmic features with abundant vacuolated cytoplasm. The nuclei are typically enlarged and hyperchromatic, and may protrude into the glandular lumen resulting in a hobnail appearance. The nuclei may also be smudged or optically clear. Mitoses are usually rare or absent.

Arias-Stella reaction can be differentiated from clear cell adenocarcinoma (Figs. 38.4, 38.5, 38.6) by the following: (1) clinical history of pregnancy—a diagnosis of adenocarcinoma clear cell type should be made with caution in a pregnant woman and should be associated with a mass and histologic examination that shows carcinoma; (2) associated decidual change in the cervix near the glands showing Arias-Stellar reaction; (3) the papillary tufting pattern, when present, is uniform in size and shape and regularly spaced instead of erratic; (4) the nuclei tend to be dark and homogeneous—most of the cells lack nuclear pleomorphism and prominent nucleoli; (5) mitotic activity is rarely present; and (6) there is no gross evidence suggestive of tumor and no stromal invasion.

PROGNOSIS AND TREATMENT

ARC in the cervix occurs during pregnancy and is an example of benign atypia that is not of clinical relevance.

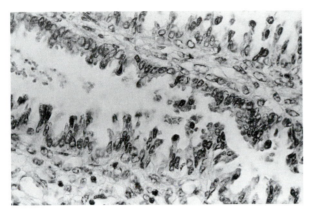

Figure 38.1. Cervical-Arias-Stella reaction.

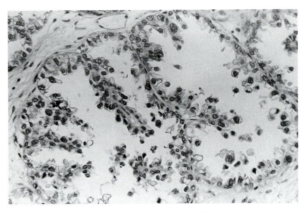

Figure 38.2. Cervical-Arias-Stella reaction.

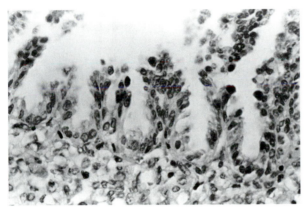

Figure 38.3. Cervical-Arias-Stella reaction.

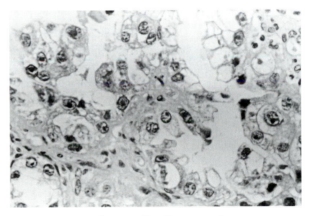

Figure 38.4. Clear cell adenocarcinoma.

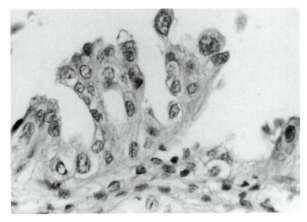

Figure 38.5. Clear cell adenocarcinoma.

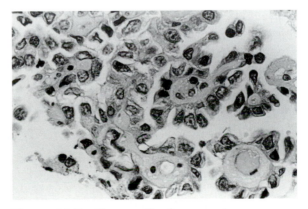

Figure 38.6. Clear cell adenocarcinoma.

39. Mesonephric Remnants

vs.

Mesonephric Hyperplasia

vs.

Mesonephric Carcinoma

CLINICAL

Mesonephric remnants and hyperplasia are found in ≤22% of adult cervices and in ≤40% of those in newborns and children. There is, however, wide variation in their frequency, which is largely dependent on extent and site of sampling. The patients usually range in age from 21 to 72 years, with a mean age of 37 years. Mesonephric remnants and hyperplasia are always asymptomatic incidental findings detected on either cervical biopsy, cone biopsy, or hysterectomy specimens that have been removed for unrelated reasons. Mesonephric carcinomas are extremely rare, and only a few cases have been reported. The patients have ranged in age from 34 to 71 years, with a mean age of 43 years. The patients may present with abnormal bleeding or may be asymptomatic, and the adenocarcinoma may be detected during investigation for unrelated symptoms.

GROSS

Mesonephric remnants and hyperplasia do not produce any gross abnormalities. Mesonephric remnants run parallel to the long axis of the uterus and in the cervix are located in the stroma of the lateral walls of the endocervix. Sections that include the lateral walls of the cervix are much more likely to include mesonephric remnants.

The few cases of mesonephric carcinoma that have been described have not shown any gross abnormalities or slight induration without a mass.

HISTOLOGY

Mesonephric remnants consist of small tubules or cysts that are located deep in the lateral cervix wall (Fig. 39.1). The tubules are arranged in small clusters or often have a main branch or duct with smaller tubules clustered in lobules around it. The tubules are lined by a single layer of nonciliated low-columnar to cuboidal or flattened epithelium. The linning cells contain no mucin or glycogen and are nonciliated. The tubular lumen, however, often contains inspissated intraluminal pink homogeneous material that is periodic acid–Schiff (PAS)-positive. Mitotic figures are rare or absent. These tubules lack connection with the surface epithelium. A prominent basement membrane may surround the tubules. The remnants may undergo cystic dilatation. Squamous metaplasia rarely occurs in these cystic structures.

Mesonephric remnants may exhibit florid hyperplasia that have been designated as lobular mesonephric hyperplasia, diffuse mesonephric hyperplasia, and mesonephric duct hyperplasia (Fig. 39.2). The division between lesions classified as mesonephric remnant and those designated mesonephric hyperplasia is often arbitrary. A diagnosis of hyperplasia is based on the presence of a prominent proliferation of tubules, an increase in lobule size, more irregularities in shape, and the diffuse, often full-thickness involvement of the cervix, often distinct from the central duct. Lobular mesonephric hyperplasia is characterized by the retention of the lobular organization despite the marked proliferation of the tubules (Fig. 39.3). The tubules vary from small round to oval to curved or branched and are occasionally dilated. Characteristically, they contain bright pink, PAS-positive hyaline material in their lumens. Lobular hyperplasia tends to occur at a younger age than in diffuse hyperplasia and is smaller in extent but deeper in the cervical stroma at its most superficial aspect. In diffuse hyperplasia, no lobular grouping is apparent and the hyperplasia is not restricted to the lateral aspects of the cervix but may be present in sections from all quadrants (Fig. 39.4). In both types of mesonephric hyperplasia the cells may show mild variation in cell size and shape and more variation in staining intensity of the cytoplasm. The cuboidal to columnar cells lining the tubules occasionally form small papillary tufts, and rare mitotic figures may be noted.

The rarest form of mesonephric hyperplasia is pure ductal hyperplasia in which a dilated, large, elongated duct, unassociated with endocervical clefts, is lined by pseudostratified epithelium that often forms small papillary tufting. These ducts resemble those seen focally in cases of lobular or diffuse hyperplasia; however, the tubules may be absent.

Mesonephric adenocarcinoma usually arises deep in the lateral wall of the cervix, in a site corresponding to the location of mesonephric remnants. The histologic features of mesonephric carcinoma are variable and are dependent on the degree of differentiation (Figs. 39.5, 39.6). In general, the predominant pattern is that of tubules and glands that are usually closely packed or may be separated by stroma. They are usually small and round, but occasionally may undergo cystic dilatation. The cells lining these tubules are cuboidal or columnar. The cytoplasm may contain scant amounts of glycogen but not mucicarmine. The lumens typically contain bright pink or red hyaline PAS-positive material. Increased crowding, confluence, and even a solid component with prominent mitotic figures may be observed in moderately and poorly differentiated forms. The tumors usually extensively invade the cervical wall in a haphazard fashion. A desmoplastic reaction is usually absent; however, the surrounding stroma may show a mild inflammatory response. Tumors with a malignant spindle cell component (malignant mesonephric mixed tumors) have been described. The surface endocervical mucosa is usually uninvolved; however, the tumor sometimes may erode into it. Mesonephric adenocarcinoma can be differentiated from mesonephric hyperplasia by the infiltrative pattern of growth, back-to-back arrangement of glands, and the presence of nuclear atypia, necrosis, and a desmoplastic stromal response. Mesonephric hyperplasia is, however, often present at the periphery of the mesonephric adenocarcinoma; however, transition between the two lesions may be extremely difficult to demonstrate.

PROGNOSIS AND TREATMENT

Mesonephric hyperplasia of all degrees appears to have a benign biologic behavior. Long-term follow-up, however, is not available, and diffuse hyperplasia or hyperplasia with any significant degree of cytologic or architectural atypia may warrant clinical follow-up. Mesonephric adenocarcinomas are extremely rare, and experience with their prognosis and treatment is limited to a few case reports.

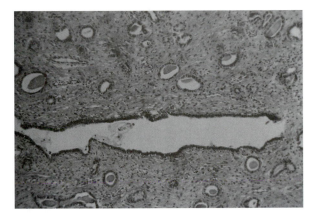

Figure 39.1. Mesonephnic remnants

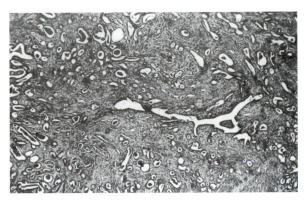

Figure 39.2. Mesonephnic hyperplasia. type.

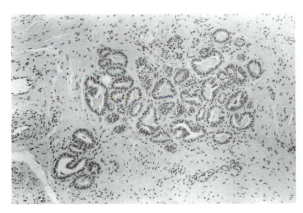

Figure 39.3. Mesonephnic hyperplasia lobular

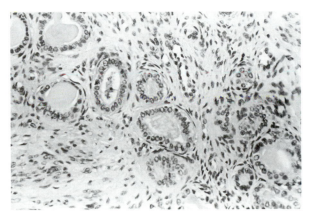

Figure 39.4. Mesonephnic hyperplasia, diffuse type.

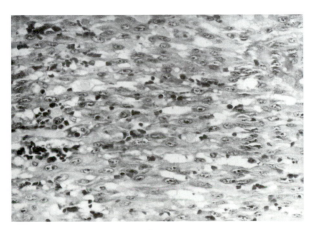

Figure 39.5. Mesonephnic carcinoma.

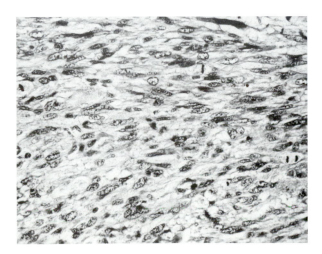

Figure 39.6. Mesonephnic carcinoma.

40. Adenoid Basal Cell Carcinoma

vs.

Adenoid Cystic Carcinoma

CLINICAL

Adenoid basal carcinoma usually occurs in postmenopausal women in the 4th to 7th decades, with the average age of ≈ 60 years. It has a high frequency in black patients. Most patients are asymptomatic, and the lesion is usually an unexpected incidental finding at cone biopsy or hysterectomy performed for coexisting CIN.

Adenoid cystic carcinoma of the cervix is exceedingly rare. It usually occurs in elderly, often multigravida, black patients in the 6th and 7th decades. Only 5% of patients are 40 years or younger. Patients usually present with abnormal uterine bleeding. It is relatively commonly associated with synchronous mucinous or other epithelial tumors of the ovary.

GROSS

The cervix in adenoid basal carcinoma usually is normal on pelvic and gross examination or shows mild nodular distortion.

Adenoid cystic carcinoma may present an irregular hard nodular exophytic or infiltrating endophytic cervical mass, often with surface ulceration.

HISTOLOGY

Adenoid basal cell carcinomas are usually composed of organoid lobules and small nests or cords of small round to oval cells with a peripheral palisaded arrangement resembling basal cell carcinoma of the skin with squamous differentiation (Fig. 40.1). The cells have a scant rim of cytoplasm and small uniform oval hyperchromatic nuclei (Fig. 40.2). Nucleoli are inconspicuous, and mitotic activity is low, usually with 0–1 mitotic figures per nest. Foci of squamous differentiation commonly occur centrally with the squamous cells with a layer of palisading smaller rounded basal cells at the periphery (Fig. 40.3).Occasionally, cells may contain eosinophilic cytoplasm, suggesting individual cell keratinization. The cell nests may also contain small lumina. Characteristically, there is no or minimal stromal response. Vascular lymphatic invasion is not seen. Approximately 50% of tu-

mors also coexist with in situ or invasive adenocarcinoma with mucous secretion. An association or direct continuity from the basal layer of dysplastic squamous epithelium, carcinoma in situ, or early invasive squamous cell carcinoma has been reported.

The histologic pattern of adenoid cystic carcinoma varies with the degree of differentiation. A tubular pattern predominates in the well-differentiated tumors, whereas a solid nesting growth is characteristic of poorly differentiated neoplasms. The morphologic appearance is similar to that observed in the more common salivary gland location of adenoid cystic carcinoma (Fig. 40.4). The tumor is composed of small, uniform cells that invade in sheets, clusters, cords, and trabeculae (Fig. 40.5). Most tumors have the distinctive cribriform pattern in which small basaloid cells form microcysts that may be empty or contain basophilic mucinous substance or eosinophilic hyaline material. There is usually at least focal palisading of cells at the periphery of the cylindromatous structures.

The nuclei adenoid cystic carcinoma are small, dark, and relatively uniform and seldom show pleomorphism. Mitotic figures are usually frequent. Hyalinization of the stroma, focal myxoid change, or fibroblastic proliferation may be prominent. Lymphatic invasion is often present; however, nerve sheath invasion is uncommon. In about half of the cases, squames or glandular differentiation may be observed at the center of tumor nests. Less frequently, malignant squamous cells form solid nests indistinguishable from squamous cell carcinoma (Fig. 40.6). The central glandular or cystic spaces may be filled with necrotic debris. An unusual case of cervical carcinosarcoma with an adenoid cystic carcinomatous component has been reported. Adenoid cystic carcinoma may also be associated with an overlying CIN, which may be responsible for the occasional abnormal cytologic smears.

ANCILLARY STUDIES

Unlike adenoid cystic carcinomas in other locations, immunostains for actin and S-100 stains for myoepithelial cells are negative in most adenoid cystic carcinomas of the cervix. The cells rarely demonstrate myoepithelial differentiation by electron microscopy.

TREATMENT AND BEHAVIOR

Adenoid basal carcinoma has a favorable prognosis. Metastases has not been reported in patients whose tumors have the typical microscopic pattern. Treatment of adenoid basal carcinoma has been hysterectomy because of its deep location in most instances. The tumor, however, may present as an incidental finding in a hysterectomy specimen removed for other reasons. Conization may be appropriate under certain circumstances.

Adenoid cystic carcinoma has a poorer prognosis than conventional squamous cell carcinoma. These neoplasms are usually deeply infiltrative, tend to recur, and often metastasize to lung and less commonly bone, liver, and brain. Radiotherapy may be suboptimal, and radical hysterectomy with lymph node dissection may be justified.

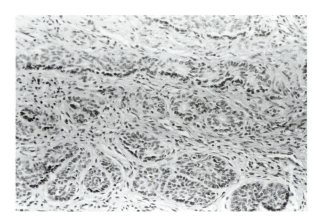

Figure 40.1. Adenoid basal cell carcinoma.

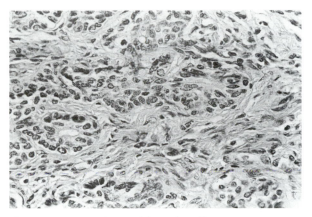

Figure 40.2. Adenoid basal cell carcinoma.

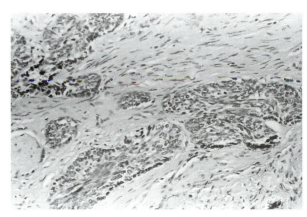

Figure 40.3. Adenoid basal cell carcinoma.

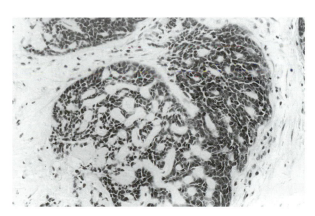

Figure 40.4. Adenoid cystic carcinoma.

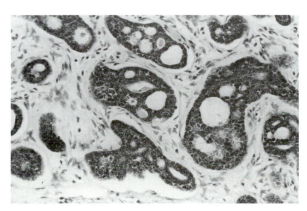

Figure 40.5. Adenoid cystic carcinoma.

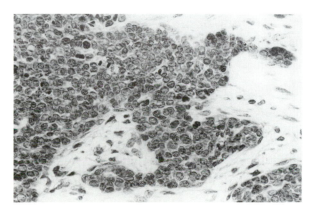

Figure 40.6. Adenoid cystic carcinoma.

41. Cervical Lymphoma

vs.

Lymphoepithelioma-like Carcinoma

CLINICAL

Malignant lymphoma may involve the cervix either as a primary tumor or, more frequently, secondarily in the course of systemic widespread disease. At autopsy approximately 1–5% of women with lymphoma have involvement of the cervix. Patients with cervical lymphoma range in age from 15 to 90 years with a mean age, as per various studies, of 41–44 years. Patients with granulocytic sarcoma of the cervix range in age from 32 to 71 years with a mean age of 50 years. The clinical presentation of cervical lymphoma does not differ from that of other more common primary tumors. The presenting complaints are usually vaginal bleeding and vaginal discharge, sometimes accompanied by pain. Occasionally a patient with lymphoma may be asymptomatic. Patients with generalized lymphoma have, in addition, anemia, splenomegaly, and others signs of lymphoma at the time of diagnosis.

Lymphoepithelioma-like carcinoma represents approximately 5.5% of cervical carcinoma. It has a definite apparent propensity for younger patients, and slightly more than half the patients are under the age of 40. The presenting symptoms are similar to those of other types of cervical carcinoma.

GROSS

Lymphomas of the cervix may result in a diffuse, barrel-shape, or multinodular polypoid enlargement of the cervix. Lymphomas may also present as a polypoid endocervical mass protruding through the cervical os. Least commonly, the cervix has a granular, ragged, or reddened surface as a result of ulceration of the tumor. Local extension of the tumor into the vagina, paracervical tissues, or lower uterine corpus is common. The cut surface is usually white to tan, homogeneous, and rubbery to firm. Granulocytic sarcomas may have similar appearance or have a green to gray-blue color when freshly cut, giving rise to the term chloroma.

Lymphoepithelioma-like carcinoma usually presents as a well-defined mass that often shows superficial ulceration and a bulging homogeneous grayish-white solid cut surface.

HISTOLOGY

Lymphomas and leukemic infiltration of the cervix may produce follicular (nodular) or diffuse patterns (Figs. 41.1, 41.2, 41.3). The histologic diagnosis depends on the malignant character of the lymphoid cells. The neoplastic cells are usually monomorphic, cytologically atypical, and mitotically active (Fig. 41.2). The most common lymphoma is diffuse large cell "histiocytic" lymphoma. The overlying epithelium is rarely infiltrated, and there is usually a thin collagenous zone immediately subjacent to the surface squamous epithelium. Lymphomas tend to deeply invade the cervical wall. Perivascular infiltration is more often observed with nodular lymphomas. Sclerosis may be prominent and result in the neoplastic cells being arranged in an epithelial-like pattern of nests or cords separated by abundant fibrous stroma (Fig. 41.1). In addition, the sclerotic areas may contain large clear lymphoid cells that became spindle-shaped causing a resemblance of the lymphoma to a sarcoma. An infiltrate of small lymphocytes and, often, plasma cells is frequently present immediately beneath the epithelium and at the periphery of the lymphomatous infiltrates. Ulceration, hemorrhage, and necrosis are rare.

Histologically lymphoepithelioma-like carcinomas are identical to the lymphoepitheliomas that occur in nasopharynx (nasopharyngeal carcinoma), salivary glands, breasts, and thymus (Fig. 41.4). They tend to be well circumscribed and composed of solid nests and cords of undifferentiated cells with indistinct cell borders (syncytium) surrounded by a marked inflammatory infiltrate (Fig. 41.5). The tumor cells are large, polygonal, and uniform in size and shape and have abundant clear to eosinophilic granular cytoplasm. Their nuclei are large and round to oval, display uniformity in shape, and have a vesicular chromatin pattern with one or more nucleoli (Fig. 41.6). Mitotic figures may be numerous. They do not demonstrate evidence of keratinization or glandular differentiation. The inflammatory component is reactive and consists of eosinophils, plasma, and lymphocytes and is present not only in the stroma but also inside the tumor parenchyma. This neoplasm has been variously described as inflammatory carcinoma, cervical carcinoma with marked lymphocytic inflammation, and circumscribed carcinoma with marked lymphocytic–eosinophilic infiltrate. No significant desmoplastic reaction is present in the supporting stroma.

In most cases of lymphoepithelioma-like carcinoma, the epithelial nature of lymphoepithelioma-like carcinoma is readily apparent; however, in cases where the malignant cells are widely separated in inflammatory stroma, the neoplasm could be mistaken for lymphoma. Immunoperoxidase staining for keratin and leukocyte common antigen have been shown to be helpful in this differentiation.

PROGNOSIS AND TREATMENT

Follicular lymphomas and diffuse large cell lymphomas with cytoplasmic clearing present more often as localized disease and have a better prognosis than nonclear and immunoblastic lymphomas. The stage of the disease is, however, the most important single factor in predict-ing survival. Cervical lymphomas can be treated by hysterectomy, usually combined with postoperative radiation, chemotherapy, or both. When the lymphoma is localized to the cervix, approximately 90% of patient survive 5 years or more. When the lymphoma involves pelvic lymph nodes or ovaries, the chance of survival decreases to 20%. Prior to making therapeutic decisions, it is important to appreciate that lymphomas originating in the genital tract are very rare compared to involvement by systemic lymphoma, and staging investigations must be thorough.

Lymphoepithelioma-like carcinoma appears to have a relatively favorable prognosis. The incidence of lymph node metastases is significantly lower than that for usual types of squamous cell carcinoma, and consequently the 5-year survival rates are significantly better. Clinical stage is an important prognostic factor as it is for other cervical tumors. Radiation appears to be effective in eradication of localized low-stage disease.

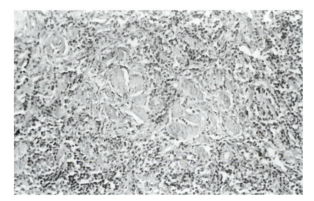

Figure 41.1. Cervical lymphoma with desmoplastic response.

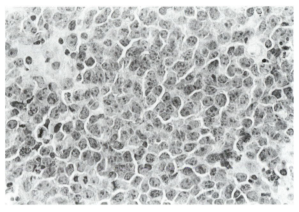

Figure 41.2. Cervical lymphoma, diffuse large cell type.

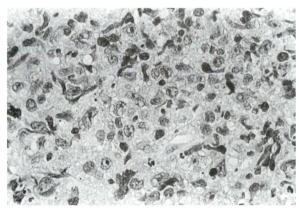

Figure 41.3. Cervical lymphoma, diffuse large cell type.

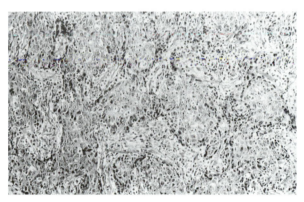

Figure 41.4. Lymphoepithelioma-like carcinoma.

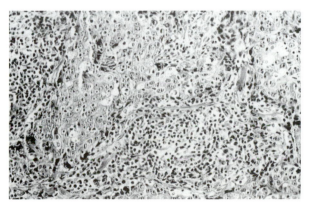

Figure 41.5. Lymphoepithelioma-like carcinoma.

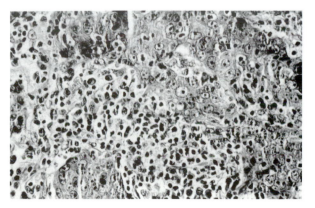

Figure 41.6. Lymphoepithelioma-like carcinoma.

42. Cervical Lymphoma
vs.
Pseudolymphoma

CLINICAL

The clinical features of cervical lymphoma are presented in Chapter 41.

Inflammatory lesions of the cervix are seldom so extensive and florid as to cause confusion with lympho-proliferative neoplasms. These lesions have been variably referred to as *lymphoma-like,* or *pseudolymphoma.* The patients are usually in the reproductive age group with an average age of 35 years. Presenting symptoms include vaginal discharge or bleeding, sometimes post-coital. One reported patient presented with nocturnal fever and was subsequently diagnosed as having infectious mononucleosis. Occasionally, patients are asymptomatic and investigated because of an abnormal cytologic smear.

GROSS

In most patients the cervix is described as soft, focally eroded or ulcerated, nodular, and friable. Rarely, these lesions present as large, exophytic masses. In some patients, the cervix is normal. In contrast, patients with cervical lymphoma have a barrel-shaped cervix or multinodular polypoid enlargement of the cervix, and mucosal ulceration is rare (Figs. 42.1, 42.2, 42.3). In addition, lymphomas frequently extend into paracervical tissue or the vagina.

HISTOLOGY

Lymphoma-like lesions are composed of a polymorphic, band-like superficial infiltrate that rarely extends below the level of the endocervical clefts (Fig. 42.4). The lymphoid infiltrate is usually diffuse and less often mixed diffuse and nodular. It consists of large lymphoid cells (centroblasts and immunoblasts), admixed with mature lymphocytes, plasma cells, and neurophils (Figs. 42.5, 42.6). Mitotic activity may be brisk. The infiltrate commonly includes germinal centers and macrophages. In contrast to cervical lymphoma, lymphoma-like lesions usually extend to the mucosa, and mucosal ulceration is common. Stromal sclerosis and perivascular infiltration are seldom seen. Close packing of follicles, absence of mantelzone, lack of starry sky pattern, and the presence of cleaved lymphoid cells between follicles favor nodular lymphoma over follicular cervicitis.

PROGNOSIS AND TREATMENT

Lymphoma-like lesions are benign, and clinical follow-up is usually uneventful. Accurate distinction between lymphoma-like lesions and lymphoma is essential to avoid errors that have important therapeutic implications. A biopsy that reveals an atypical but nondiagnostic lymphoid infiltrate should be followed by a large incisional or excisional biopsy. Immunohistochemical and molecular diagnostic studies may be employed to assist in the diagnosis.

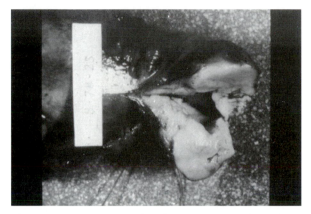

Figure 42.1. Cervical enlargement in lymphoma.

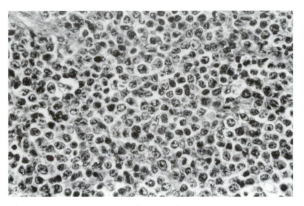

Figure 42.2. Cervical lymphoma monotonous infiltrate of abnormal large cells.

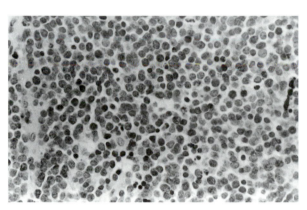

Figure 42.3. Cervical lymphoma.

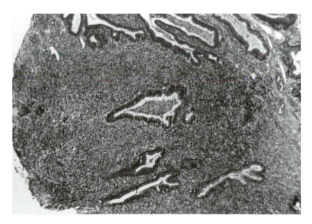

Figure 42.4. Lymphoid infiltrate involving endocervix.

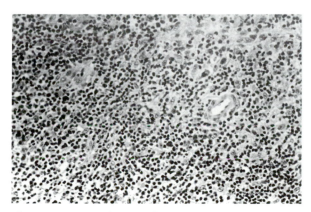

Figure 42.5. Polymorphic population of lymphocytes and histiocytes characteristic of pseudolymphoma.

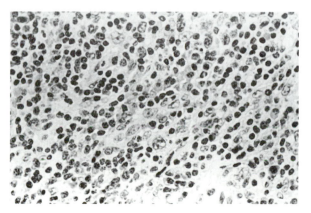

Figure 42.6. Lymphoma-like reactive infiltrate.

Section 4 BIBLIOGRAPHY AND INDEX

Bibliography

Chapter 1

Hewitt J. Histological criteria for lichen sclerosus of the vulva. J Reprod Med 31:781–787, 1986.

Lawrence WD. Non-neoplastic epithelial disorders of the vulva (vulvar dystrophies): Historical and current perspectives. In Pathology Annual, Rosen PP, Fechner RE (eds), Appleton & Lange. Part II, vol 28:23–51, 1993.

Pincus SH, Stadecker MJ. Vulvar dystrophies and noninfectious inflammatory conditions. In: Wilkinson EJ (eds) Contemporary issues in surgical pathology. Pathology of the Vulva and Vagina, vol. 9, New York, Churchill Livingstone, 11–24, 1987.

Ridley CM. The vulva. Philadelphia, WB Saunders 1975.

Chapter 2

Kurman RJ, Norris HJ, Wilkinson E. Tumors of the cervix, vagina, and vulva. Atlas of Tumor Pathology, Third Series, Fascicle 4, Washington, D.C., Armed Forces Institute of Pathology, 1992.

Lawrence WD. Non-neoplastic epithelial disorders of the vulva (vulvar dystrophies): Historical and current perspectives. In Pathology Annual, Rosen PP, Fechner RE (eds), Appleton & Lange. Part II, vol 28:23–51, 1993.

Pincus SH, Stadecker MJ. Vulvar dystrophies and noninfectious inflammatory conditions. In: Wilkinson EJ (eds) Contemporary issues in surgical pathology. Pathology of the Vulva and Vagina. New York, Churchill Livingstone, vol 9:11–24, 1987.

Wilkinson EJ. Benign diseases of the vulva. In: Kurman RJ (ed) Blaustein's Pathology of the Female Genital Tract, 4th ed. New York, Springer-Verlag, 31–86, 1994.

Wilkinson EJ. Premalignant and malignant tumors of the vulva. In: Kurman RJ (ed) Blaustein's Pathology of the Female Genital Tract, 4th ed. New York, Springer-Verlag, 87–129, 1994.

Chapter 3

Dodson RF, Fritz GS, Hubler WR, Rudolph AH, Knox JM, Chu LW. Donovanosis: a morphologic study. J Invest Dermatol 62:611–614, 1974.

Douglas CP. Lymphogranuloma venereum and granuloma inguinale of the vulva. J Obstet Gynecol Br Commun 69:871–880, 1962.

Kurman RJ, Norris HJ, Wilkinson E. Tumors of the cervix, vagina, and vulva. Atlas of Tumor Pathology, Third Series, Fascicle 4, Washington, D.C., Armed Forces Institute of Pathology, 1992.

Sehgal VN, Shyamprasad AL, Beohar PC. The histopathological diagnosis of donovanosis. Br J Vener Dis 60:45–47, 1984.

Chapter 4

Kurman RJ, Potkul RK, Lancaster WD, Lewandowski G, Weck PR, Delgato G. Vulvar condylomas and squamous vestibular micropapilloma: differences in appearance and response to treatment. J Reprod Med 35:1019–1022, 1990.

Majmudar B, Castellano PZ, Wilson RW, Siegel RJ. Granular cell tumors of the vulva. J Reprod Med 35:1008–1014, 1990.

Wilkinson EJ. Premalignant and malignant tumors of the vulva. In: Kurman RJ (ed) Blaustein's Pathology of the Female Genital Tract, 4th ed. New York, Springer-Verlag, 87–129, 1994.

Wolber RA, Talerman A, Wilkinson EJ, Clement PB. Vulvar granular cell tumors with pseudocarcinomatous hyperplasia: a comparative analysis with well-differentiated squamous carcinoma. Int J Gynecol Pathol 10:59–66, 1991.

Chapter 5

Kurman RJ, Norris HJ, Wilkinson E. Tumors of the cervix, vagina, and vulva. Atlas of Tumor Pathology, Third Series, Fascicle 4, Washington, D.C., Armed Forces Institute of Pathology, 1992.

Wade TR, Kopf AW, Ackerman AB. Bowenoid papulosis of the penis. Cancer 42:1890–1903, 1978.

Wade TR, Kopf AW, Ackerman AB. Bowenoid papulosis of the genitalia. Arch Dermatol 115:306–308, 1979.

Wilkinson EJ. Premalignant and malignant tumors of the vulva. In: Kurman RJ (ed) Blaustein's Pathology of the Female Genital Tract, 4th ed. New York, Springer-Verlag, 87–129, 1994.

Chapter 6

Bacci CE, Goldfogel GA, Greer BE, Gown AM. Paget's disease and melanoma of the vulva. Use of a panel of monoclonal antibodies to identify cell type and to microscopically define adequacy of surgical margins. Gynecol Oncol 46:216–221, 1992.

Benda JA, Platz CE, Anderson B. Malignant melanoma of the vulva: a clinical-pathologic view of 16 cases. Int J Gynecol Pathol 5:202–216, 1986.

Gunn RA, Gallager HS. Vulvar Paget's disease: a topographic study. Cancer 46:590–594, 1980.

Michael H, Roth LM. Paget's disease, skin appendage tumors, and congenital and acquired cysts of the vulva. In Wilkinson EJ (ed) Pathology of the vulva and vagina, vol. 9. New York, Churchill Livingstone, 25–48, 1987.

Nadji M, Ganjei P. The application of immunoperoxidase techniques in the evaluation of vulvar and vaginal disease. In: Wilkinson EJ (ed) Contemporary issues in surgical pathology. Pathology of the vulva and vagina, vol. 9. New York, Churchill Livingstone, 239–248, 1987.

Pierson KK. Maligant melanomas and pigmented lesions of the vulva. In: Wilkinson EJ (ed) Contemporary issues in surgical pathology. Pathology of the vulva and vagina, vol. 9. New York, Churchill Livingstone, 155–179, 1987.

Tasseron EW, van der Esch EP, Hart AA, Brutel de la Riviere G, Aartsen EJ. A clinicopathological study of 30 melanomas of the vulva. Gynecol Oncol 46:170–175, 1992.

Toker C. Clear cells of the nipple epidermis. Cancer 25 (3):601–610, 1970.

Chapter 7

Christensen WN, Friedman KJ, Woodruff JD, Hood AF. Histologic characteristics of vulvar nevocellular nevi. J Cutan Pathol 14:87–91, 1987.

Friedman RJ, Ackerman B. Difficulties in the histologic diagnosis of melanocytic nevi on the vulvae of pre-menopausal women. In: Ackerman AB (eds) Pathology of malignant mela-noma. New York, Mason, 119–127, 1981.

Pierson KK. Maligant melanomas and pigmented lesions of the vulva. In: Wilkinson EJ (ed) Contemporary issues in surgical pathology. Pathology of the vulva and vagina, vol. 9. New York, Churchill Livingstone, 155–179, 1987.

Rhodes AR, Mihm MC Jr, Weinstock MA. Dysplastic melanocytic nevi. A reproducible histologic definition emphasizing cellular morphology. Mod Pathol 2:306–319, 1989.

Chapter 8

Bergeron C, Ferenczy A, Richart RM, Guralnick M. Micropapillomatosis labialis appears unrelated to human papillomavirus. Obstet Gynecol 76:182–286, 1990.

Campion MJ, Dipaola FM, Crozier MA, Rathrock R, Vellios F, Franklin EW. Labial micropapillomatosis human papillomavirus infection or anatomic variant. Obstet Gynecol 00:00-00, 1994 (In Press).

Lynch PJ. Condylomata acuminata (anogenital warts). Clinical Obstet Gynecol 28:142–151, 1985.

Moyal-Barracco M, Leibowitzh M, Orth G. Vestibular papillae of the vulva. Lack of evidence for human papillomavirus etiology. Arch Dermatol 126:1594–1598, 1990.

Oriel JD. Natural history of genital warts. Br J Vener Dis 47:1–13, 1971.

Wang AC, Hsu JJ, Hseuh S, Sun CF, Tsao KC. Evidence of human papillomavirus deoxyribonucleic acid in vulvar squamous papillomatosis. Int J Gynecol Pathol 10:44–50, 1991.

Wilkinson EJ. Benign diseases of the vulva. In: Kurman RJ (ed) Blaustein's Pathology of the Female Genital Tract, 4th ed. New York, Springer-Verlag, 31–86, 1994.

Chapter 9

Brisigotti M, Moreno A, Murcia C, Matias-Guiu X, Prat J. Verrucous carcinoma of the vulva. A clinicopathologic and imunohistochemical study of five cases. Int J Gynecol Pathol 8:1–7, 1989.

Japaze H, vanDinh T, Woodruff JD. Verrucous carcinoma of the vulva: study of 24 cases. Obstet Gynecol 60:462–466, 1982.

Kluzak TR, Krause FT. Condylomata, papillomas and verrucous carcinomas of the vulva and vagina. In: Wilkinson EJ, (ed) Pathology of the vulva and vagina. New York: Churchill Livingstone, 49–77, 1987.

Kraus FT, Perez-Mesa C. Verrucous carcinoma. Cancer 19:26–38, 1966.

Kurman RJ, Toki T, Schiffman MH. Basaloid and warty carcinomas of the vulva. Distinctive types of squamous cell carcinoma frequently associated with HPV. Am J Surg Pathol 17:133–145, 1993.

Okagaki T. Warty carcinoma of the vulva: a probable implication of human papillomavirus as the causative agent. Lab Invest 44:49A, 1981.

Rhatigan RM, Nuss RC. Keratoacanthoma of the vulva. Gynecol Oncol 21:118–123, 1985.

Shafeek MA, Osman ME, Hussein MA. Carcinoma of the vulva arising in condylomata acuminata. Obstet Gynecol 54:120–123, 1979.

Toki T, Kurman RJ, Park JS, Kessis T, Daniel RW, Shah KV. Probable nonpapillomavirus etiology of squamous cell carcinoma of the vulva in older women: a clinicopathologic study using in situ hybridization and polymerase chain reaction. Int J Gynecol Pathol 10:107–125, 1991.

Chapter 10

Abell MR. Adenocystic (pseudoadenomatous) basal cell carcinoma of vestibular glands of vulva. Am J Obstet Gynecol 86:470–482, 1963.

Addison A, Parker RT. Adenoid cystic carcinoma of Bartholin's gland. Gynecol Oncol 5:196–201, 1977.

Bernstein SG, Voet RL, Lifshitz S, Buchsbaum HJ. Adenoid cystic carcinoma of Bartholin's gland. Case report and review of the literature. Am J Obstet Gynecol 147:385–390, 1983.

Breen JL, Neubecker RD, Greenwald E, Gregori CA. Basal cell carcinoma of the vulva. Obstet Gynecol 46:122–129, 1975.

Cruz-Jimenez PR, Abell MR. Cutaneous basal cell carcinoma of the vulva. Obstet Gynecol 36:1860–1868, 1975.

Chapter 11

Freedman SR, Goldman RL. Mucocele-like changes in Bartholin's glands. Hum Pathol 9:111–114, 1978.

Junaid TA, Thomas SM. Cysts of the vulva and vagina: a comparative study. Int J Gynecol Obstet 19:239–241, 1981.

Kucera PR, Glazer J. Hydrocele of the canal of nuck: a report of four cases. J Reprod Med 30:439–442, 1985.

Marquette GP, Su B, Woodruff JD. Introital adenosis associated with Stevens-Johnson Syndrome. Obstet Gynecol 66:143–145, 1985.

Oi RH, Munn R. Mucous cysts of the vulvar vestibule. Hum Pathol 13:584–586, 1982.

Rabbi SJ, Ross JS, Prat J, Keh PC, Welch WR. Urogenital sinus origin of mucinous and ciliated cysts of the vulva. Obstet Gynecol 51:347–351, 1978.

Sedlacek TV, Riva JM, Magen AB, Mangan CE, Cunnane MF. Vaginal and vulvar adenosis. An unsuspected side-effect of CO_2 laser vaporization. J Reprod Med 35:995–1001, 1990.

Chapter 12

Lever WF, Schaumburg-Lever G. Histopathology of the skin, 6th ed. Philadelphia, JP Lippincott, 1990.

Mann MS, Kaufman RH. Erosive lichen planus of the vulva. Clin Obstet Gynecol 34:605–613, 1991.

Pelisse M. The vulva-vaginal-gingival syndrome. A new form of erosive lichen planus. Int J Dermatol 28:381–384, 1989.

Ridley CM. The vulva. Philadelphia, WB Saunders, 1975.

Wilkinson EJ. Benign diseases of the vulva. In: Kurman RJ (ed) Blaustein's Pathology of the Female Genital Tract, 4th ed. New York, Springer-Verlag, 31–86, 1994.

Chapter 13

Kneale BL. Carcinoma of the vulva then and now. The 1987 ISSVD presidential address. J Reprod Med 33:454–456, 1988.

Mene A, Buckley CH. Involvement of the vulval skin appendages by intraepithelial neoplasia. Br J Obstet Gynecol 92:634–638, 1985.

Shatz P, Bergeron C, Wilkinson EJ, Arseneau J, Ferenczy A. Vulvar intraepithelial neoplasia and skin appendage involvement. Obstet Gynecol 74:769–774, 1989.

Wilkinson EJ. Superficially invasive carcinoma of the vulva. Clin Obstet Gynecol 34:651–661, 1991.

Wilkinson EJ. Superficially invasive carcinoma of the vulva. In: Wilkinson EJ (ed) Contemporary issues in surgical pathology. Pathology of the vulva and vagina, vol 9. New York, Churchill Livingstone, 103–117, 1987.

Chapter 14

Gad A, Eusebi V. Rhabdomyoma of the vagina. J Pathol 115: 179–181, 1975.

Gold JH, Bossen EH. Benign vaginal rhabdomyoma. A light and electron microscopic study. Cancer 37:2283–2294, 1976.

Hilgers RD, Malkasian GD Jr. Soule EH. Embryonal rhabdomyosarcoma (botryoid type) of the vagina: a clinicopathologic review. Am J Obstet Gynecol 107:484–502, 1970.

Newton WA, Soule EH, Hamoudi AB, et al. Histopathology of childhood sarcomas, intergroup rhabdomyosarcoma studies I and II: clinicopathologic correlation. J Clin Oncol 6:67–75, 1988.

Tsokos M, Webber BL, Parham DM, et al. Rhabdomyosarcoma. A new classification scheme related to prognosis. Arch Pathol Lab Med 116:847–855, 1992.

Chapter 15

Begin LR, Clement PB, Kirk ME, Jothy S, McCaughey WT, Ferenczy A. Aggressive angiomyxoma of pelvic soft parts: a clinicopathologic study of nine cases. Hum Pathol 16:621–628, 1985.

Cheung TH, Chan MK, Chang A. Aggressive angiomyxoma of the female perineum: case reports. Aust N Z J Obstet Gynaecol 31:285–287, 1991.

Miettinen M, Wahlstrom T, Vesterinen E, Saksela E. Vaginal polyps with pseudosarcomatous features. A clinico-pathologic study of seven cases. Cancer 51:1148–1151, 1983.

Mucitelli DR, Charles EZ, Kraus FT. Vulvovaginal polyps. Histologic appearance, ultrastructure, immunocytochemical characteristics of clinicopathologic correlations. Int J Gynecol Pathol 9:20–40, 1990.

Norris HJ, Taylor HB. Polyps of the vagina. A benign lesion resembling sarcoma botryoides. Cancer 19:227–232, 1966.

Ostor AG, Fortune DW, Riley CB. Fibroepithelial polyps with atypical stromal cells (Pseudosarcoma botryoides) of vulva and vagina. A report of 13 cases. Int J Gynecol Pathol 7:351–360. 1988.

Steeper TA, Rosai J. Aggressive angiomyxoma of the female pelvis and perineum. Report of nine cases. Am J Surg Pathol 7:463–475, 1983.

Chapter 16

Silverberg SG, Frable WJ. Prolapse of fallopian tube into vaginal vault after hysterectomy. Histopathology, cytopathology, and differential diagnosis. Arch Pathol 97:100–103, 1974.

Ulbright TM, Alexander RW, Kraus FT. Intramural papilloma of the vagina: evidence of Mullerian histogenesis. Cancer 48: 2260–2266, 1981.

Wheelock JB, Schneider V, Goplerud DR. Prolapsed fallopian tube masquerading as adenocarcinoma of the vagina in a postmenopausal woman. Gynecol Oncol 21:369–375, 1985.

Chapter 17

Guillou L, Gloor E, DeGrandi P, Costa J. Post-operative pseudosarcoma of the vagina. A case report. Pathol Res Pract 185:245–248, 1989.

Peters WA, Kumar NB, Anderson WA, Morley GW. Primary sarcoma of the adult vagina: a clinicopathologic study. Obstet Gynecol 65:699–704, 1985.

Proppe KH, Scully RE, Rosai J. Postoperative spindle cell nodules of genitourinary tract resembling sarcomas. A report of eight cases. Am J Surg Pathol 8:101–108, 1984.

Tavassoili FA, Norris HJ. Smooth muscle tumors of the vagina. Obstet Gynecol 53:689–693, 1979.

Young RH, Scully RE. Pseudosarcomatous lesions of the urinary bladder, prostate gland, and urethra. A report of three cases and review of the literature. Arch Pathol Lab Med 111:354–358, 1987.

Chapter 18

Branton PA, Tavassoli FA. Spindle cell epithelioma, the so-called mixed tumor of the vagina. Am J Surg Path 17:509–515, 1993.

Buntine DW, Henderson PR, Biggs JSG. Benign mullerian mixed tumor of the vagina. Gynecol Oncol 21–26, 1979.

Sirota RL, Dickerson GR, Scully RE. Mixed tumors of the vagina: a clinicopathologic analysis of eight cases. Am J Surg Pathol 5:413–422, 1981.

Steeper TA, Piscioli F, and Rosai J. Squamous cell carcinoma with sarcoma-like stroma of the female genital tract. Clinicopathologic study of four cases. Cancer 52:890–898, 1983.

Chapter 19

Fu YS, Reagan JW. Pathology of the uterine cervix, vagina, and vulva, Chapter 7. Philadelphia, WB Saunders, 193–224, 1989.

Gallup DG, Morley GW. Carcinoma in situ of the vagina: a study and review. Obstet Gynecol 46:334, 1975.

Gray LA, Christopherson MM. In-situ and early invasive carcinoma of the vagina. Obstet Gynecol 34:226, 1969.

Kaufman RH, Friedrich EG, Gardner HL. Cystic tumors. In: Benign disease of vulva and vagina, 3rd ed, Chapter 9. Chicago, Year Book Medical Publishers, 237–285, 1989.

Chapter 20

Friedrich EG, Siegesmund KA. Tampon-associated vaginal ulcerations. Obstet Gynecol 55:149–156, 1980.

Gardner HL. Desquamative inflammatory vaginitis: a newly defined entity. Am J Obstet Gynecol 102:1102–1105, 1968.

Jimerson SD, Becker JD. Vaginal ulcers associated with tampon usage. Obstet Gynecol 56:97–99, 1980.

Kaufman RH, Friedrich EG, Gardne HL. Atrophic, desquamative, and postradiation vulvovaginitis. In: Benign diseases of the vulva and vagina, 3rd ed, Chapter 16. Chicago, Year Book Medical Publishers, 419–434, 1989.

McCormack WM. Unusual vulvovaginal conditions: Interstitial cystitis, focal vulvitis and desquamative inflammatory vaginitis. In: Sobel JD (ed) Vulvovaginal infections: Current concepts in diagnosis and therapy. New York, Academy Professional Information Services, Inc., 149–160, 1990.

Pelisse M. The vulva-vaginal-gingival syndrome. A new form of erosive lichen planus. Int J Dermatol 28:381–384, 1989.

Chapter 21

Antonioli Da, Burke L, Friedman EA. Natural history of diethylstibestrol-associated genital lesions: cervical ectopy and cervicovaginal hood. Am J Obstet Gynecol 137:847–853, 1980.

Noller KL, Townsend DE, Kaufman RH, et al. Maturation of vaginal and cervical epithelium in women exposed in utero to diethylstilbestrol (DESAD Project). Am J Obstet Gynecol 146:279–285, 1983.

Robboy SJ, Hill EC, Sandberg EC, Czernobilsky B. Vaginal adenosis in women born prior to the diethylstilbestrol (DES) era. Hum Pathol 17:488–492, 1986.

Robboy SJ, Young RH, Welch WR, et al. Atypical (dysplastic) adenosis: forerunner and transitional state to clear cell adenocarcinoma in young women exposed in utero to diethylstilbestrol. Cancer 54:869–875, 1984.

Zaino RJ, Robboy SJ, Bentley R, Kurman RJ. Diseases of the vagina. In: Kurman RJ (ed) Blaustein's Pathology of the Female Genital Tract, 4th ed. New York, Springer-Verlag, 131–183, 1994.

Chapter 22

Herbst AL, Anderson S, Hubby MM, et al. Risk factors for the development of diethylstibestrol-associated clear cell adenocarcinoma: a case-control study. Am J Obstet Gynecol 154:814–822, 1986.

Herbst AL, Ulfelder H, Poskanzer DC. Adenocarcinoma of the vagina: association of maternal stilbestrol therapy with tumor appearance in young women. N Engl J Med 284:878–881, 1971.

Robboy SJ, Szyfelbein WM, Goellner JR, et al. Dysplasia and cytologic findings in 4,589 young women enrolled in diethylstibestrol-adenosis (DESAD) project. Am J Obstet Gynecol 140:579–586, 1981.

Robboy SJ, Welch WR, Young RH, et al. Topographic relation of adenosis, clear cell adenocarcinoma and other related lesions of the vagina and cervix in DES-exposed progeny. Obstet Gynecol 60:546–551, 1982.

Robboy SJ, Young RH, Welch WR, et al. Atypical vaginal adenosis and cervical ectropion. Association with clear cell adenocarcinoma in diethylstilbestrol-exposed offspring. Cancer 54:869–875, 1984.

Zaino RJ, Robboy SJ, Bentley R, Kurman RJ. Diseases of the vagina. In: Kurman RJ (ed) Blaustein's Pathology of the Female Genital Tract, 4th ed. New York, Springer-Verlag, 131–183, 1994. C:\WPWIN60\WPDOCS\CEM\FINALREF.097

Bibliography For Section 3

General References

Anderson MC: The pathology of cervical cancer. Clin Obstet Gynecol 12:87/119, 1985.

Clement PB: Miscellaneous Primary Tumors and Metastatic Tumours of the Uterine Cervix. In Obstetrical and Gynecological Pathology. Fox H and Wells M ed. New York, NY Churchill Livingstone, 1995, p 345.

Crum CP, Nuovo GJ: The Cervix. In Diagnostic Surgical Pathology. Ed 2. Sternberg SS, ed. New York, Raven Press, 1994, p 2055.

Fu YS, Reagan JW: Pathology of the Uterine Cervix, Vagina, and Vulva, Philadelphia, W.B. Saunders, 1989, p225.

Gompel C, Silverberg SG: The cervix. In Pathology in Gynecology and Obstetrics, ed. 4. Philadelphia, J.B. Lippincott, 1994, p72.

Kraus F: Female Genitalia. In Anderson's Pathology, ed. 9. St. Louis, C.V. Mosby Company, Kissane JM, ed 1990, p1620.

Kurman RJ, Norris HJ, Wilkinson EW: Atlas of tumor pathology: tumors of the cervix, vagina, and vulva. Washington, DC, AFIP, 1992, p7.

Lawrence D: Advances in the pathology of the uterine cervix. Hum Pathol 22: 802/806, 1991.

Robert ME, Fu YS: Squamous cell carcinoma of the uterine cervix: a review with emphasis on prognostic factors and unusual variants. Semin Diagn Pathol 7:173/189, 1990.

Rosai J: Uterus-cervix. In Ackerman's Surgical Pathology, ed 7. St. Louis, C.V. Mosby Company, 1996, p1353.

Woodruff JD, Augtuaco TL, Parmley TH: The Cervix. In Atlas of Gynecologic Pathology, ed 2. New York, Raven Press, 1993.

Zaloudek C: The vulva, vagina and cervix. In: The Difficult Diagnosis in Surgical Pathology. Philadelphia, PA. W.B. Saunders Company, Weidner N, ed, 1996, p534.

Chapter 23

Ambros RA, Kurman RJ: Current concepts in the relationship of human Papilloma virus infection to the pathogenesis and classification of pancancerous squamous lesions of the uterine cervix. Semin Diagn Pathol 7:158/172, 1990.

Kurman RJ, Henson DE, Herbst AL, et al: Interim guidelines for management of abnormal cervical cytology. JAMA 271: 1866/1869, 1994.

Nelson JH, Averette HE, Richart RM: Cervical intraepithelial neoplasia (dysplasia and carcinoma in situ) and early invasive cervical carcinoma. CA Cancer J Clin 39:157/178, 1989.

Schiffman, Brinton LA: The epidemiology of cervical carcinogenesis. Cancer 76:888/901, 1995.

Wright TC, Kurman RJ, Ferenczy A: Precancerous Lesions of the Cervix. In Blaustein's Blaustein's Pathology of the Female Genital Tract, ed. 4. New York, Springer-Verlag (Kurman RJ, ed), 1994, p229.

Chapter 24

See General References

Albores-Saavedra J, Young RH: Transitional cell neoplasm (carcinomas and inverted papillomas) of the uterine cervix. A report of five cases. Am J Surg Pathol 19:1138/1145, 1995.

Chapter 25

Yelverton CL, Bentley RC, Olenick S, et al: Epithelial report of the uterine cervix: Assessment of morphologic features and correlations with cytologic diagnosis. Int J Gynecol Pathol 15:338/344, 1996.

Chapter 26

See General References.

Boon ME, van Dunne FMF, Vardaxis NJ: Ideas in Pathology. Recognition of atypical reserve cell hyperplasia in cervical smears and its diagnostic significance. Mod Pathol 8:786/794, 1995.

Chapter 27

See General References.

Jovanic AS, McLachlin CM, Shen L, et al: Postmenopausal squamous atypia: a spectrum including pseudokoilocytosis. Mod Pathol 8:408/412, 1995.

Prasad CJ, Sheets E, Selig AM, et al: The binucleate squamous cell: histologic spectrum and relationship to low-grade squamous intraepithelial lesions. Mod Pathol 6:313/317, 1993.

Chapter 28

Creasman WT: Editorial. New gynecologic cancer staging. Gynecol Oncol 58:157/158, 1995.

Larsson G, Alm P, Bullberg B, et al: Prognostic factors in early invasive carcinoma of the uterine cervix. Am J Obstet Gynecol 146:145/152, 1983.

Robert ME, Fu YS: Squamous cell carcinoma of the uterine cervix. A review with emphasis on prognostic factors and unusual variants. Semin Diagn Pathol 7:173/189, 1990.

Selvaggi SM: Cytologic features of squamous cell carcinoma in situ involving endocervical glands in endocervical cytobrush specimens. Acta Cytol 38:687/692, 1994.

Seven B-U, Nadji M, Averette HE, et al: Microinvasive carcinoma of the cervix. Cancer 70:2121/2128, 1992.

Van Nagel JR, Greenwell N, Powell DF: Microinvasive carcinoma of the cervix. Am J Obstet Gynecol 145:981/991, 1983.

Chapter 29

Maier RC, Norris HJ: Glassy cell carcinoma of the cervix. Obstet Gynecol 60:219/224, 1982.

Tamimi HK, Ek M, Hesla J, et al: Glassy cell carcinoma of the cervix redefined. Obstet Gynecol 71:837/841, 1988.

Chapter 30

Armenia CS, Shaver DN, Modisher MW: Decidual transformation of the cervical stroma simulating reticulum cell sarcoma. Am J Obstet Gynecol 89:808/816, 1964.

Bausch RG, Kaump DH, Alles RW: Observations of the decidual reaction of the cervix during pregnancy. Am J Obstet Gynecol 58:777/783, 1949.

Clement PB, Young RH, Scully RE: Nontrophoblastic pathology of the female genital tract and peritoneum associated with pregnancy. Semin Diagn Pathol 6:372/406, 1989.

Huettner PC, Gersell DJ: Placental site nodule: A clinicopathologic study of 38 cases. Int J Gynecol Pathol 13:191/198, 1994.

Tsukamoto N, Nakamura M, Kashimura M: Primary cervical choriocarcinoma. Gynecol Oncol 9:99/107, 1980.

Young RH, Kurman RJ, Scully RE: Placental site nodules and plaques: A clinicopathologic analysis of 20 cases. Am J Surg Pathol 14:1001/1009, 1990.

Young RH, Kurman RJ, Scully RE: Proliferations and tumors of intermediate trophoblast of the placental site. Semin Diagn Pathol 5:223/237, 1988.

Zaytsev P, Taxy JB: Pregnancy-associated ectopic decidua. Am J Surg Pathol 11:526/530, 1987.

Chapter 31

Ambros RA, Park J, Shah KV, et al: Evaluation of histologic, morphometric, and immunohistochemical criteria in the differential diagnosis of small cell carcinomas of the cervix with particular reference to human Papilloma virus types 16 and 18. Mod Pathol 4:586/593, 1991.

Barrett RJ, Davos I, Leuchter RS, et al: Neuroendocrine features in poorly differentiated and undifferentiated carcinomas of the cervix. Cancer 60:2325/2330, 1987.

Gersell DJ, Mazoujian G, Mutch DG, et al: Small cell undifferentiated carcinoma of the cervix. Am J Surg Pathol 12:684/698, 1988.

Silva EG, Gershenson D, Sneige N, et al: Small cell carcinoma of the uterine cervix: pathology and prognostic factors. Surg Pathol 2:105/115, 1989.

Silva EG, Kott MM, Ordonez NG: Endocrine carcinoma intermediate cell type of the uterine cervix. Cancer 54:1705/1713, 1984.

Chapter 32

Clement PB, Young RH, Scully RE: Stromal endometriosis of the uterine cervix: A variant of endometriosis that may stimulate a sarcoma. Am J Surg Pathol 14:449/455, 1990.

Novotny DB, Maygarden SJ, Johnson DE: Tubal metaplasia. A frequent potential pitfall in the cytologic diagnosis and endocervical glandular dysplasia on cervical smears. Acta Cytol 36:1/10, 1992.

Rosen PP, Fechner RE: Pathology of endometriosis. Pathol Annu 25:245/295, 1990.

Suh K, Silverberg SG: Tubal metaplasia of the uterine cervix. Int J Gynecol Pathol 9:122/128, 1990.

Chapter 33

Jaworski RC, Pacey NF, Greenberg ML: The histologic diagnosis of adenocarcinoma in situ and related lesions of the cervix uteri. Cancer 61:1171/1181, 1988.

Kaspar HG, Dinh TV, Doherty MG, et al: Clinical implications of tumor volume measurement in stage I adenocarcinoma of the cervix. Obstet Gynecol 81:296–300, 1993.

Chapter 34

See General References.

Gloor E. Hurlimann J: Cervical intraepithelial glandular neoplasia (adenocarcinoma in situ and glandular dysplasia). Cancer 58:1272/1280, 1986.

Griffin NR, Wells M: Premalignant and malignant glandular lesions of the cervix. In Obstetrical and Gynecological Pathology. New York, NY Churchill Livingstone, Fox H and Wells M, eds. 1995, p323.

Hitchcock A, Johnson J, McDowell K, et al: A retrospective study into the occurrence of cervical glandular atypia in cone biopsy specimens from 1977-1978 with clinical follow-up. Int J Cancer 3:164/168, 1993.

Fluhmann CF: Focal hyperplasia (tunnel clusters) of the cervix uteri. Obstet Gynecol 17:206/214, 1961.

Gilks CB, Young RH, Aguirre P, et al: Benign endometrial adenomyomas and adenoma malignum. Mod Pathol 9:220/224, 1996.

Jones MA, Young RH: Endocervical type A (noncystic) tunnel clusters with cytologic atypia: A report of 14 cases. Am J Surg Pathol 20:1312/1318, 1996.

McGowan L, Young RH, Scully RE: Peutz-Jeghers syndrome with adenoma malignum of the cervix: A report of two cases. Gynecol Oncol 10:125/133, 1980.

McKelvey JL, Goodlin RR: Adenoma malignum of the cervix: A cancer of deceptively innocent histological pattern. Cancer 16:549/557, 1963.

Michael H, Grawe L, Kraus FT: Minimal deviation endocervical adenocarcinoma: Clinical and histologic features, immunohistochemical staining for carcinoembryonic antigen, and differentiation from confusing benign lesions. Int J Gynecol Pathol 3:261/276, 1984.

Segal GH, Hart WR: Cystic endocervical tunnel clusters: A clinicopathologic study of 29 cases of so-called adenomatous hyperplasia. Am J Surg Pathol 14:895/903, 1990.

Silverberg SG, Hurt WG: Minimal deviation adenocarcinoma (adenoma malignum) of the cervix: A reappraisal. Am J Obstet Gynecol 121:971/975, 1975.

Steeper TA, Wick MR: Minimal deviation adenocarcinoma of the uterine cervix (adenoma malignum). Cancer 58:1131/1138, 1986.

Chapter 36

Gilks CB, Clement PB: Papillary serous adenocarcinoma of the uterine cervix: A report of three cases. Mod Pathol 5:426/431, 1992.

Hopson L, Jones MA, Boyce CR: Papillary villoglandular carcinoma of the cervix. Gynecol Oncol 39:221/224, 1990.

Jones MW, Silverberg SB, Kurman RJ: Well-differentiated villoglandular adenocarcinoma of the uterine cervix: A clinicopathological study of 24 cases. Int J Gynecol Pathol 12:1/7, 1993.

Rose PG, Reale FR: Serous papillary carcinoma of the cervix. Gynecol Oncol 50:361/364, 1993.

Young RH, Scully RE: Villoglandular papillary adenocarcinoma of the uterine cervix: A clinicopathologic analysis of 13 cases. Cancer 63:1773/1779, 1989.

Young RH, Scully RE: Invasive adenocarcinoma and related tumors of the uterine cervix. Semin Diagn Pathol Vol 7, No 3, 1190, pp205/227.

Chapter 37

Clement PB, Young RH, Scully RE: Nontrophoblastic pathology of the female genital tract and peritoneum associated with pregnancy. Semin Diagn Pathol 6:372/406, 1989.

Kyriakos M, Kempson RL, Konikov NF: A clinical and pathologic study of endocervical lesions associated with oral contraceptives. Cancer 22:99/110, 1968.

Leslie KO, Silverberg SG: microglandular hyperplasia of the cervix: unusual clinical and pathological presentations and their differential diagnosis. Progr Surg Pathol 5:95/114, 1984.

Speers WC, Picaso LG, Silverberg SG: Immunohistochemical localization of carcinoembryonic antigen in microglandular hyperplasia and adenocarcinoma of the endocervix. Am J Clin Pathol 79:105/107, 1983.

Taylor HB, Irey NS, Norris HJ: Atypical endocervical hyperplasia in women taking oral contraceptives. JAMA 202:185/187, 1967.

Young RH, Scully RE: Atypical forms of microglandular hyperplasia of the cervix simulating carcinoma. Am J Surg Pathol 13:50/56, 1989.

Young RH, Scully RE: Uterine carcinomas simulating microglandular hyperplasia. A report of six cases. Am J Surg Pathol 16:1092/1097, 1992.

Young RH, Clement PB: Pseudoneoplastic glandular lesions of the uterine cervix. Semin Diagn Pathol Vol 8, No 4, 1991, pp234/249.

Young RH, Scully RE: Invasive adenocarcinoma and related tumors of the uterine cervix. Semin Diagn Pathol Vol 7, No 3, 1190, pp205/227.

Chapter 38

Cove H: The Arias-Stella reaction occurring in the endocervix in pregnancy: recognition and comparison with an adenocarcinoma of the endocervix. Am J Surg Pathol 3:567/568, 1979.

Chapter 39

Clement PB, Young RH, Keh P, et al: Malignant mesonephric neoplasms of the uterine cervix. Am J Surg Pathol 19:1158/1171, 1995.

Clement PB, Young RH, Keh P, et al: Malignant mesonephric neoplasms of the uterine cervix. Am J Surg Pathol 19:1158/1171, 1995.

Ferry JA, Scully RE: Mesonephric remnants, hyperplasia, and neoplasia in the uterine cervix. Am J Surg Pathol 14:1100/1111,1990.

Hart WR, Norris HJ: Mesonephric adenocarcinomas of the cervix. Cancer 29:106/113, 1972.

Seidman JD, Tavassoli FA: Mesonephric hyperplasia of the uterine cervix. A clinicopathologic study of 51 cases. Int J Gynecol Pathol 14:293/299, 1995.

Stewart CRJ, Taggart CR, Brett F, et al: Mesonephric adenocarcinoma of the uterine cervix with focal endocrine cell differentiation. Int J Gynecol Pathol 112:264/269, 1993.

Young RH, Scully RE: Invasive adenocarcinoma and related tumors of the uterine cervix. Semin Diagn Pathol 7:205/227, 1990.

Chapter 40

Ferry JA, Scully RE: Adenoid cystic carcinoma and adenoid basal carcinoma of the uterine cervix: a study of 28 cases. Am J Surg Pathol 12:134/144, 1988.

Hoskins WJ, Averette HE, Ng APB, et al: Adenoid cystic carcinoma of the cervix uteri: report of 6 cases and review of the literature. Gynecol Oncol 7:371/384, 1979.

Manhoff DT, Schiffman R, Haupt HM: Adenoid cystic carcinoma of the uterine cervix with malignant stroma: an unusual variant of carcinosarcoma? Am J Surg Pathol 19:229/323, 1995.

Mazure MT, Battifora HA: Adenoid cystic carcinoma of the uterine cervix: Ultrastructure, immunofluorescence, and criteria for diagnosis. Am J Clin Pathol 77:494/500, 1982.

Chapter 41

Haliz MA, Kragel PJCT: Carcinoma of the uterine cervix resembling lymphoepithelioma. Obstet Gynecol 66:829,831, 1985.

Hasumi K, Sugano H, Sakamoto G, et al: Circumscribed carcinoma of the uterine cervix, with marked lymphocytic infiltration. Cancer 39:2503,2507, 1977.

Kapp DS, LiVolsi VA: Intense eosinophilic stromal infiltration in carcinoma of the uterine cervix: A clinicopathologic study of 14 cases. Gynecol Oncol 16:19/30, 1983.

Ladefoged C, Lorentzen M: Xanthogranulomatous inflammation of the female tract. Histopathology 13:541/551, 1988.

Meis JM, Butler JJ, Osborne BM, et al: Granulocytic sarcoma in nonleukemic patients. Cancer 58:2697/2709, 1986.

Mills SE, Austin MB, Randall ME: Lymphoepithelioma-like carcinoma of the uterine cervix: A distinctive, undifferentiated carcinoma with inflammatory stroma. Am J Surg Pathol 9:884/889, 1985.

Perren T, Farrant M, McCarthy K, et al: Lymphomas of the cervix and upper vagina: a report of five cases and a review of the literature. Gynecol Oncol 44:87/95, 1992.

Chapter 42

Young RH, Harris NL, Scully RE: Lymphoma-like lesions of the lower female genital tract: a report of 16 cases. Int J Gynecol Pathol 4:289/299, 1985.

INDEX

References in *italics* denote figures